DEJA REVIEW™

Behavioral Science

Notice

DEJA REVIEW™

Behavioral Science

Fatima Cody Stanford, MPH

Medical College of Georgia School of Medicine
Class of 2007

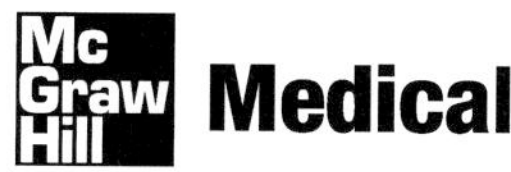

New York Chicago San Francisco Lisbon London Madrid Mexico City
Milan New Delhi San Juan Seoul Singapore Sydney Toronto

The McGraw-Hill Companies

Deja Review™: Behavioral Science

1 2 3 4 5 6 7 8 9 0 DOC/DOC 0 9 8 7 6

ISBN-10: 0-07-146868-4
ISBN-13: 978-0-07-146868-8

This book was set in Palatino by International Typesetting and Composition.

The editors were Marsha Loeb and Patrick Carr.

The production supervisor was Catherine Saggese.

The text was designed by Marsha Cohen/Parallelogram.

Project management was provided by International Typesetting and Composition.

RR Donnelley was printer and binder.

This book is printed on acid-free paper.

INTERNATIONAL EDITION ISBN-10: 0-07-110091-1; ISBN-13: 978-0-07-110091-5

Library of Congress Cataloging-in-Publication Data

Stanford, Fatima Cody.
Behavioral science / Fatima Cody Stanford.
p. cm. — (Deja review)
ISBN 0-07-146868-4
1. Psychology—Examinations, questions, etc. 2. Behavioral science—Examinations, questions, etc. 3. Medicine and psychology—Examinations, questions, etc. I. Title. II. Series.

R726.5.S73 2006
616.890076—dc22

2006044852

Now unto him that is able to do exceeding abundantly above all that we ask or think, according to the power that worketh in us,
Unto him be glory in the church by Christ Jesus throughout all ages, world without end. A-men.
—Ephesians 3:20–21

To my loving husband, my soul mate, and my joy, Corey J. Stanford, thank you for being the most supportive person ever and for the wonderful diagrams that you provided for the text.
To my father, mother, and sister, thank you for believing in me and contributing to my overall well-being.
To my church family at the Church of the Abiding Presence Truth and Teaching Center, thank you for guiding me to lead a life by faith, and teaching me to operate in kingdom of God authority as I strive to do the greater works and exceed them as I abide in the Spirit's presence for both guidance and manifestation.
To my extended family and friends, thanks for your encouragement.
To my countless mentors, thanks for helping me to push for the highest possible level of achievement.

And this is the confidence that we have in him, that, if we ask any thing according to his will, he heareth us:
And if we know that he hear us, whatsoever we ask, we know that we have the petitions that we desired of him.
—I John 5: 14–15

Contents

Faculty Reviewers

Josephine Albritton, MD
Director, Psychiatry Clerkship
Medical College of Georgia School of Medicine
Augusta, Georgia

Sean Blitzstein, MD
Director, Psychiatry Clerkship
Clinical Assistant Professor of Psychiatry
University of Illinois at Chicago School of Medicine
Chicago, Illinois

Donna Londino, MD
Assistant Professor, Psychiatry and Health Behavior
Child Adolescent and Family Psychiatry
Medical College of Georgia School of Medicine
Augusta, Georgia

Carol A. Schwab, JD, LLM.
Assistant Dean for Legal/Medical Education
Professor in the Department of Psychiatry and Health Behavior
Medical College of Georgia School of Medicine
Augusta, Georgia

Student Reviewers

Silke Heinisch
Medical Student
Temple University Medical School
Class of 2007

Alicia K. Morgans
Medical Student
University of Pennsylvania School of Medicine
Class of 2006

Contributing Authors

Saima Arshad
Class of 2007
Medical College of Georgia School of Medicine
Augusta, Georgia

Jenifer Dye
Class of 2007
Medical College of Georgia School of Medicine
Augusta, Georgia

Stephanie A. Freeman
Class of 2006
University of Kentucky School of Medicine
Lexington, Kentucky

Alinda P. Gary, MD
Resident, Psychiatry & Behavioral Science
Baylor College of Medicine
Houston, Texas

Melanie Hafford
Class of 2007
Medical College of Georgia School of Medicine
Augusta, Georgia

Janet Hickey, MD
Resident, Psychiatry & Behavioral Science
Baylor College of Medicine
Houston, Texas

Kasha Otway James
Class of 2007
Howard University School of Medicine
Washington, District of Columbia

Barbara Semakula
Class of 2007
Loma Linda School of Medicine
Loma Linda, California

Sherri Simpson, MD
Resident, Psychiatry & Behavioral Science
Baylor College of Medicine
Houston, Texas

Alfredo Bellon Velasco, MD
Resident, Psychiatry & Behavioral Science
Baylor College of Medicine
Houston, Texas

Gie Na Yu
Class of 2007
Medical College of Georgia School of Medicine
Augusta, Georgia

Preface

Step 1 of the United States Medical Licensing Exam (USMLE) tests the sophomore medical student's ability to apply the core principles of the basic sciences. In order to accomplish this feat, you must be able to recall a vast amount of information. The *Deja Review* series is the most efficient, well-organized, portable, and high yield resource to prepare students for the USMLE. As a medical student who recently took Step 1, I am confident that I have compiled a novel review guide that promotes rapid recall of all of the essential facts necessary for success on the behavioral science portion of the examination. Often, students do not spend a considerable time preparing for the behavioral science section since they feel as though these questions are the "easy" questions. Yet, students do not perform any better on the behavioral science section than the other sections of the test. Students should devote their time to getting the most questions correct, regardless of their level of difficulty. This book sets out to help you ace the behavioral science portion of the exam.

ORGANIZATION

All concepts are presented in a question and answer format that covers the key facts on numerous behavioral science topics. The material is divided into chapters covering the major topics in behavioral science. I have also included topics on legal issues in medicine, epidemiology, and biostatistics.

The question and answer format has several important advantages:

- It provides a rapid, straightforward way for you to assess your strengths and weaknesses.
- It allows you to efficiently review and commit to memory a large body of information.
- If offers you a break from tedious, convoluted multiple choice questions.
- The clinical vignettes will expose you to the prototypic presentation of behavioral science topics classically tested on the USMLE Step 1.
- It serves as a quick, last minute review of high yield facts.

HOW TO USE THIS BOOK

Remember, this text is not intended to replace comprehensive textbooks, course packs, or lectures. It is, however, intended to serve as a supplement to your studies during the first and second years of medical school. This text has been sampled by a number of medical students who found it to be an essential part of their preparation for the USMLE Behavioral Science shelf examination, in addition to Step 1 itself. Begin using this book early in your first year of medical school. You may cover up the answers to quiz yourself and your fellow classmates. For a greater challenge, try covering up the questions!

However you choose to study, we hope you find this resource helpful during your preparation for the USMLE Step 1 and throughout your basic science years. I pray for your success!

Fatima Cody Stanford, MPH

Acknowledgments

I would like to thank all of the contributors and faculty reviewers for their invaluable contributions to this text and their efforts to make this a useful resource for students.

I would like to thank Fred Rose of McGraw-Hill who recommended me as a potential writer to the McGraw-Hill editors. Finally, I would like to thank Marsha Loeb, my editor, who was there with me every step of the way as we brought this book into fruition.

CHAPTER 1

The Early Stages of Life: Infancy to Adolescence

THEORIES OF DEVELOPMENT

Name four developmental theorists.

Erik Erikson

Sigmund Freud

Margaret Mahler

Jean Piaget

Describe Erik Erikson's theories of development.

Critical periods at which achievement of social goals need to be achieved, otherwise they won't be achieved.

Describe Sigmund Freud's theories of development.

Parts of the body from which pleasure is derived at each age of development.

Describe Margaret Mahler's theories of development.

Early development is a sequential process of separation of the child from the mother or primary care provider.

Describe Jean Piaget's theories of development.

Learning capabilities of the child at various ages during development; children must move through four stages of development. There is a specific set of skills that must be mastered at each stage of development before progression to the other stages.

Erik Erikson's Theory of Development

Which stage of development is characterized by an infant establishing faith in their caregiver?	Trust vs. Mistrust present from birth to 18 months
Which stage of development is characterized by a child learning physical skills such as walking and learning to use the bathroom?	Autonomy vs. Shame and Doubt present from age 18 months to 3 years
Which stage of development is characterized by a child becoming assertive in their learning?	Initiative vs. Guilt present from age 3 to 6 years
Which stage of development is characterized by a child acquiring new skills at a rapid rate?	Industry vs. Inferiority present from age 6 to 12 years
Which stage of development is characterized by a teen who achieves a sense of identity in politics, sex roles, or occupation?	Identity vs. Role Confusion present from age 12 to 18 years
Which stage of development is characterized by an adult determining whether or not they want to establish an intimate relationship with another individual?	Intimacy vs. Isolation present from age 19 to 40 years
Which stage of development is characterized by an adult finding ways to support and encourage the next generation?	Generativity vs. Stagnation present from age 40 to 65 years
Which stage of development is characterized by an adult reflecting on their life experience?	Ego Integrity vs. Despair present from age 65 years to death

Sigmund Freud's Theory of Development

Which stage of development is characterized by focus on receiving pleasure through food consumption or sucking on pacifiers?	Oral phase present from birth to age 1 year
Which stage of development is characterized by focus on receiving pleasure through potty training?	Anal phase present from age 1 to 3 years

Which stage of development is characterized by focus on identifying with adult role models and the oedipal complex?

Phallic phase present from age 3 to 6 years

Which stage of development is characterized by focus on expanding social interactions?

Latency phase present from age 6 to 12 years

Which stage of development is characterized by focus on establishing a family?

Genital phase present from age 13 to adulthood

Margaret Mahler's Theories of Development

Which stage of development is characterized by an infant trying to achieve homeostasis with the environment?

Normal autistic phase from birth to 4 weeks

Which stage of development is characterized by an infant becoming aware of their environment and identifying with their care taker?

Normal symbiotic phase from age 4 weeks to 5 months

Which stage of development is characterized by an infant becoming more alert and being able to identify who is familiar vs. who is a stranger?

First subphase: Differentiation present from age 5 to 10 months

Which stage of development is characterized by an infant learning to walk?

Second subphase: Practicing present from age 10 to 16 months

Which stage of development is characterized by a toddler's frustration with his or her inability to complete a task without his/her caregiver's assistance?

Third subphase: Rapprochement present from age 16 to 24 months

Which stage of development is characterized by a toddler's acceptance of his or her caregiver's absence?

Fourth subphase: Constancy phase present from age 24 to 36 months

Jean Piaget's Theory of Development

Which stage of development is characterized by infants and toddlers focus on their eyes, ears, hands, and other senses?

Sensorimotor period from birth to 2 years

Which stage of development is characterized by children acquiring representational skills in the area of mental imagery and language?

Preoperational thought present from age 2 to 7 years

Which stage of development is characterized by children being more logical, flexible, and organized than in early childhood?

Concrete operations present from age 7 to 12 years

Which stage of development is characterized by being able to think logically, theoretically, and abstractly?

Formal operations from age 12 to adulthood

INFANT MORBIDITY AND MORTALITY

Define premature birth.

Less than *34 weeks* gestation or birth weight less than *2500 g*

What are the potential outcomes of being a premature infant?

Increased infant mortality

Delayed physical and social development

Emotional and behavioral problems

Dyslexia

Child abuse

In the United States, what percentage of births is premature?

6% for White women and 13% for African American women. An average of 7.2 per 1000 live births

What are the common risk factors associated with premature births?

Low socioeconomic status

Teenage pregnancy

Poor maternal nutrition

NEONATAL REFLEXES

What are the six important neonatal reflexes?

Moro

Palmar grasp

Rooting

Stepping

Asymmetric tonic neck

Parachute

Which are present at birth?

Moro

Palmar grasp

Rooting

Stepping

What is the Moro reflex?

Head extension causes extremity extension followed by flexion.

What is the palmar grasp?

If finger is placed in infant's palm, it is grasped.

What is the rooting reflex?

If an object is placed around an infant's mouth, the infant will pursue it.

What is the stepping reflex?

When held upright and leaning forward, an infant will make walking motions with their legs.

At what age do the Moro, palmar, rooting, and stepping reflexes disappear?

4 to 6 months

What is the asymmetric tonic neck?

While supine, turning of the head causes ipsilateral extremity extension and contralateral flexion.

At what age does it appear and then disappear?

Present at 2 weeks and disappears by 6 months

What is the parachute reflex?

While sitting and tilted to one side, an infant extends the ipsilateral arm to support the body.

DEVELOPMENTAL MILESTONES

What are the key categories of development?

Gross motor

Fine/visual motor

Language

Social

What are the developmental milestones at 1 month of age?

Gross motor: When prone lifts head slightly

Fine/visual: With eyes tracks objects to midline; tight grasp

Language: Startles to sound

Social: Fixes on face

What are the developmental milestones at 2 to 3 months of age?

Gross motor: Steadily *holds head up*; when prone lifts chest up

Fine/visual: Hands open at rest

Language: *Smiles responsively*; coos

Social: *Recognizes parents*; reaches for familiar objects or people

What are the developmental milestones at 4 to 5 months of age?

Gross motor: *Rolls* front to back and back to front; sits well supported

Fine/visual: *Grasps* with both hands

Language: Orients to voice

Social: Laughs; enjoys observing environment

What are the developmental milestones at 6 months of age?

Gross motor: *Sits* well unsupported; sits upright

Fine/visual: Transfers hand to hand; *reaches* with either hand

Language: *Babbles*

Social: Recognizes strangers and has *stranger anxiety*

What are the developmental milestones at 9 months of age?

Gross motor: Crawls, cruises, pulls to stand

Fine/visual: Uses *pincer grasp*; finger feeds

Language: Says "dada/mama;" understands "No"

Social: Waves bye-bye; plays pat-a-cake

What are the developmental milestones at 12 months of age?

Gross motor: Cruises/*walks* alone

Fine/visual: Throws, releases objects

Language: One to eight words other than "dada/mama;" one-step commands

Social: Imitates actions; comes when called; cooperates with dressing

What are the developmental milestones at 15 months of age?

Gross motor: Walks backward; creeps upstairs

Fine/visual: Builds *two-block towers*; scribbles; uses a cup

Language: Uses four to eight words

Social: Throws *temper tantrums*

What are the developmental milestones at 18 months of age?

Gross motor: Runs; kicks a ball

Fine/visual: Feeds self with utensils

Language: Points to body parts when asked; names common objects

Social: Plays around but not with other children; start of toilet training

What are the developmental milestones at 21 months of age?

Gross motor: Squats and recovers

Fine/visual: Builds *five-block towers*

Language: Two-word combinations

Social: *Toilet training*

What are the developmental milestones at 24 months of age?

Gross motor: *Walks well up and down stairs; jumps*

Fine/visual: Removes clothing; copies a line

Language: 50-word vocabulary; stranger understands half of speech

Social: Follows two-step commands; engages in *parallel play*

What are the developmental milestones at 30 months of age?

Gross motor: *Throws ball* over hand

Fine/visual: Removes clothes; copies lines

Language: Appropriate pronoun use

Social: Knows first and last names

What are the developmental milestones at 3 years of age?

Gross motor: Pedals *tricycle;* goes up and down stairs with alternating feet

Fine/visual: *Draws a circle;* eats with utensils

Language: Three-word sentences; uses plurals and past tense; stranger understands three-fourths of speech

Social: *Group play;* shares toys

What are the developmental milestones at 4 years of age?

Gross motor: *Hops and skips*

Fine/visual: Catches ball; dresses alone; *copies a cross*

Language: *Knows colors;* counts to 10

Social: *Imaginative play*

What are the developmental milestones at 5 years of age?

Gross motor: *Hops and skips*

Fine/visual: *Ties shoes*

Language: Prints first name

Social: Plays *cooperative games; understands rules* and abides by them

Table 1.1 Developmental Milestones

	Gross Motor	Fine/visual Motor	Language	Social
1 month old	When prone lifts head slightly	With eyes tracks objects to midline; tight grasp	Startles to sound	Fixes on face
2 to 3-months old	Steadily holds head up; when prone lifts chest up	Hands open at rest	Smiles responsively; coos	Recognizes parents; reaches for familiar objects or people
4 to 5-months old	Rolls front to back and back to front; sits well supported	Grasps with both hands	Orients to voice	Laughs; enjoys observing environment
6 months old	Sits well unsupported; sits upright	Transfers hand to hand; reaches with either hand	Babbles	Recognizes strangers and has stranger anxiety
9 months old	Crawls, cruises, pulls to stand	Uses pincer grasp; finger feeds	Says "dada/mama;" understands "No"	Waves bye-bye; plays pat-a-cake
12 months old	Cruises/walks alone	Throws, releases objects	One to eight words other than "dada/mama;" one-step commands	Imitates actions; comes when called; cooperates with dressing
15 months old	Walks backward; creeps upstairs	Builds two-block towers; scribbles; uses a cup	Uses four to eight words	Throws temper tantrums
18 months old	Runs; kicks a ball	Feeds self with utensils	Points to body parts when asked; names common objects	Plays around but not with other children; start of toilet training
21 months old	Squats and recovers	Builds five-block towers	Two-word combinations	Toilet training

24 months old	Walks well up and down stairs; jumps	Removes clothing; copies a line	50 word vocabulary; stranger understands half of speech	Follows two-step commands; engages in parallel play
30 months old	Throws ball over hand	Removes clothes; copies lines	Appropriate pronoun use	Knows first and last names
3 years old	Pedals tricycle; goes up and down stairs with alternating feet	Draws a circle; eats with utensils	Three-word sentences; uses plurals and past tense; stranger understands three-fourths of speech	Group play; shares toys
4 years old	Hops and skips	Catches ball; dresses alone; copies a cross	Knows colors; counts to 10	Imaginative play
5 years old	Hops and skips	Ties shoes	Prints first name	Plays cooperative games; understands rules and abides by them

ATTACHMENT

At 7 to 12 months, separation from the mother or primary care provider results in what?	Initially protests, then anaclitic depressions
What is anaclitic depression?	When an infant becomes withdrawn and unresponsive. This can lead to death if it is severe and longstanding.
What occurs without proper mothering or attachment?	Failure to thrive
What occurs during failure to thrive?	Developmental retardation Poor health and growth High death rates, even with adequate physical care
Toddlers who are hospitalized are most likely to fear what?	Separation from parents or care providers more than bodily harm or pain
In what age group is elective surgery best tolerated?	7- to 11-year olds
By age 3, how does separation from parents or care providers affect children?	Separation from parents has no long term negative effects on children. In fact, children at age 3, are able to spend significant portions of the day with other adults.
How do toddlers understand death?	It is an *incomplete understanding* of the meaning of death and the child may expect a friend, relative or pet to come back to life.
At what age do children begin to understand the concept of death?	At the age of 8 years
How do 7- to 11-year olds react to death?	They "act out," act badly at school or home (a defense mechanism).
In what age group do children begin to form relationships with other adults?	7 to 11 years
Which parent do the 7- to 11-year olds identify themselves with?	The *same sex parent*

EARLY ADOLESCENCE (11 TO 14 YEARS)

How is the start of puberty marked?

Cognitive growth and personality formation.

In girls—the onset of *menstruation*, beginning at age 11 to 12 years

In boys—the first *ejaculation*, occurring at age 13 to 14 years

How is the development through puberty measured?

By the Tanner stages

How many Tanner stages are there and what are the three categories of measurement?

There are *five* Tanner stages. The categories are male genitalia, female breasts, and pubic hair.

Define Stage I.

Males have a childhood sized penis, testes, and scrotum

Females have preadolescent breasts with elevation of the papilla only

There is no pubic hair

Define Stage II.

Males have enlargement of the testes and scrotum

Females have breast buds with elevation of breast and papilla

Pubic hair is sparse and straight with downy hair on labia/penis base

Define Stage III.

Males have penis enlargement

Females have breast and areola enlargement with single contour

Pubic hair is curled, darker, and coarse

Define Stage IV.

Males have scrotal skin darkening and rogations are present

Females have areola and papilla projection with separate contour (secondary mound)

Pubic hair is adult type hair limited to the genital area

Define Stage V.

Males have adult sized and shaped penis, testes, and scrotum

Females have mature breasts

Pubic hair is adult quantity and pattern and spreads to the thighs

Table 1.2 Tanner Stages of Development

	Male Genitalia	Female Breasts	Pubic Hair Stage
Stage I	Childhood sized penis, testes, and scrotum	Preadolescent breasts with elevation of the papilla only	Absent
Stage II	Enlargement of the testes and scrotum	Breast buds with elevation of breast and papilla	Pubic hair is sparse and straight with downy hair on labia/penis base
Stage III	Penis enlargement	Breast and areola enlargement with single contour	Pubic hair is curled, darker, and coarse
Stage IV	Scrotal skin darkening and rogations are present	Areola and papilla projection with separate contour (secondary mound)	Pubic hair is adult type hair limited to the genital area
Stage V	Adult sized and shaped penis, testes, and scrotum	Mature breasts	Pubic hair is adult quantity and pattern and spreads to the thighs

CHAPTER 2

The Middle Stages of Life: Early and Middle Adulthood

EARLY ADULTHOOD

What age range constitutes early adulthood?	20 to 40 years
What are the primary characteristics of this stage of life?	Role in society is defined Physical development peaks Sense of independence
What critical event happens at around age 30?	Period of reappraisal
Which Erikson stage is prevalent during early adulthood?	Intimacy vs. Isolation
Which life events occur during this stage?	Marriage Having children Occupation
What percentage of Americans is married by age 30?	60% to 70%
What are three emotional postpartum reactions that women suffer from?	Postpartum "blues" Major depression Postpartum psychosis
What is the percentage of women who suffer from postpartum "blues"?	33% to 50%
What are the characteristics of postpartum "blues"?	Sadness Unhappiness

How long do the symptoms of postpartum "blues" last?	Up to 1 week post delivery
What can a physician do to assist a patient with postpartum "blues"?	Support Child care advice
What is the percentage of women who suffer from postpartum major depression?	5% to 10%
What are the characteristics of postpartum major depression?	Helplessness Hopelessness Lack of joy in usual activities
When do the symptoms of postpartum major depression occur?	4 weeks after delivery
What can a physician do to assist a patient with postpartum major depression?	Antidepressant medication Frequent scheduled visits
What percentage of women suffer from postpartum psychosis?	0.1% to 0.2%
What are characteristics of postpartum psychosis?	Delusions Hallucinations Mother may harm infant
When do the symptoms of postpartum psychosis occur?	2 to 3 weeks after delivery
What can a physician do to assist a patient with postpartum psychosis?	Antipsychotic medication Hospitalization **Note:** This is a psychiatric emergency!
Which postpartum emotional reactions is considered normal?	Postpartum "blues"
At what point should adopted children be told that they are adopted?	Earliest age possible; when they understand language

MIDDLE ADULTHOOD

What age range constitutes middle adulthood?	40 to 65 years
What are the primary characteristics of this stage of life?	Power Authority
Which Erikson stage is prevalent during middle adulthood?	Generativity vs. Stagnation
What happens to men and women in their middle forties and early fifties?	*Midlife crisis*

What happens to men and women in a *midlife crisis*?	Change in work and/or marital relationship
What are common changes seen in a *midlife crisis*?	1. Change in lifestyle or profession 2. Infidelity, separation, or divorce 3. Increased use of alcohol or drugs 4. Depression
Why do people experience a *midlife crisis*?	Become aware of aging and mortality
What term describes the decrease in physiologic function that occurs in midlife?	Climacterium
What physiologic functions decrease in men?	1. Endurance 2. Muscle strength 3. Sexual performance
What major reproductive change occurs in women?	Menopause
What are the characteristics of menopause?	1. Ovaries no longer function 2. Hot flashes 3. Lack of menstrual cycles
What medical intervention has been used to treat menopause symptoms?	Estrogen replacement therapy
How long should contraceptive measures continue after the last menstrual period?	1 year

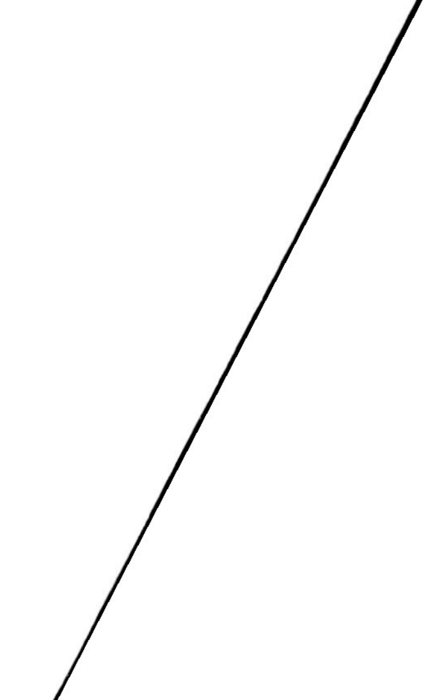

CHAPTER 3

The Late Stages of Life: Aging, Death, and Bereavement Issues

AGING

What percentage of the U.S. population will be 65 years and older by the year 2020?	15%
What is the fastest growing age group in the United States today?	85 years and older
What is the average life expectancy?	76 years
What factors within a population can have an effect on differences in life expectancy?	Gender (females tend to live longer than males; an average difference of 7 years) Race (Whites tend to live longer than Blacks) White female (80 years) > Black female (74 years) = White male (74 years) > Black male (66 years)
How are the life expectancies changing in regards to different ethnic groups?	Males and African Americans are living longer, thus the gap from the longest living (White female) is decreasing.
What physical changes are associated with aging?	Sensory: impaired vision and hearing Visceral: decreased pulmonary, renal, and gastrointestinal function Extremities: increased fat deposits, osteoporosis, decreased muscle mass and strength

What changes in the brain usually accompany aging?

Less cerebral blood flow

Decreased brain weight

Enlarged ventricles and sulci

Increased amount of senile plaques and neurofibrillary tangles (also found in older brains from patients who did not suffer from Alzheimer's disease [AD])

Psychological

Does an individual's level of intelligence change throughout life?

No (there may be less speed and forgetfulness)

What two lifestyle factors are not affected by age?

Social functioning and self-care

Which Erikson's stage of development is characteristic of the last stage of life?

Ego Integrity vs. Despair. At this point, the elderly realize that the opportunities for major life achievements (e.g., having a child) have already been accomplished. If these goals have not been obtained, there is despair for not having achieved them.

Psychopathology

What is the most common psychiatric illness of the elderly?

Depression

What factors can lead to depression in the elderly?

Loss of spouse

Loss of friends

Loss of family

Loss of prestige

Decline of health

Retirement

Loss of income

What disease process is common in the elderly population that may mimic depression and is marked by progressive memory loss and cognition problems?

Alzheimer's disease

What three methods can be used to successfully treat depression?

Pharmacotherapy

Psychotherapy

Electroconvulsive therapy (can cause anterograde and retrograde memory loss, often used if patient is refractory to other treatments)

What changes in sleep patterns occur in the elderly?

Decreased sleep quality

Less time asleep

Decreased rapid eye movement (REM) sleep

Decreased slow wave sleep

Increased sleep latency

Increased awakenings during the night

What disorder is seen in 10% to 15% of the elderly population but often unidentified?

Alcohol related disorders

Do psychiatric drugs produce the *same* effects in the elderly as they do in young adults?

No. There are differences in drug disposition and response, and the elderly have a greater susceptibility to side effects. Therefore, when you prescribe, you should *start low and go slow*.

Longevity

What factors are associated with longevity?

Family history

Continuation of occupational and physical activity

Higher education

Social support system including marriage

DYING, DEATH, AND BEREAVEMENT

Elizabeth Kubler Ross describes five stages of death and dying which usually occur in consecutive order.

At what stage would a patient refuse to believe he or she is dying and say, "You must be reading the wrong chart"?

Denial

At what stage would a patient become upset with the hospital staff and say, "You should not have kept me on those medicines for so long. That is what put me in this situation"?

Anger

At what stage would a patient plead with a higher power for forgiveness and a chance to make right whatever may be wrong in his or her life?

Bargaining

At what stage would a patient realize fighting is futile and understand and appreciate that life has come to an end?

Acceptance

What is the difference between bereavement and depression?

Bereavement is the normal grief that is experienced after a difficult situation such as losing a loved one. Depression is characterized by a persistent sad, anxious, or "empty" mood.

Note: Depressive episodes may occur after a loss.

How long does bereavement last?

The time spent in a period of bereavement depends on how attached the person was to the person who died and how much time was spent anticipating the loss.

Note: *Many* factors contribute to this, such as the nature of the relationship, other psychiatric issues/illnesses, length of the time of dying, circumstances surrounding the death, and so forth.

Table 3.1 Differences between Bereavement (Normal Grief) and Depression (Abnormal Grief)

Bereavement	Depression
Minor sleep disturbances	Major sleep disturbances
Some feelings of guilt	Feeling of worthlessness
Illusions	Hallucinations and delusions
Expressions of sadness	Suicidal thoughts and attempts
Minor weight loss (<3 lb)	Major weight loss (>8 lb)
Good grooming and hygiene	Poor grooming
Attempts to return to normal routine	Few attempts to return to normal routine
Severe symptoms subside in <2 months	Severe symptoms continue for >2 months
Moderate symptoms subside in <1 month	Moderate symptoms subside in >1 month
Tx—support groups, increased contact with physician, counseling, short-acting sedatives if needed	Tx—may include antipsychotics, electroconvulsive therapy, antidepressants, and psychotherapy

Abbreviation: Treatment, Tx.

CHAPTER 4

Psychoanalytic Theory

What are the two major theories of the mind developed by Freud?

1. Topographic theory of the mind (includes three parts):
   a. Conscious
   b. Preconscious
   c. Unconscious
2. Structural theory of the mind (also known as the tripartite theory):
   a. Ego
   b. Superego
   c. Id

Which part of Freud's topographic mind contains information that is unconscious, yet can be brought to the conscious with prompting?

The preconscious mind (just before it becomes conscious)

Which part of the mind contains thoughts a person is aware of?

The conscious—this part of the mind has no access to the unconscious. The unconscious includes what we are not aware of such as sexual drives, aggressive drives, impulses, or fantasies.

How is the expression of the id regulated?

The ego exerts the learned realities of the world over the id to control its overt expression of primitive drives, such as sexual urges and aggression. The ego manages and negotiates the drives from the id as well as the realities of the world and moral restrictions (the superego).

Which part of the mind helps a person maintain relationships?

The ego

Which part of the mind incorporates acquired moral and ethical concepts?

The superego (our *conscience*)

How does the ego deal with conflicts between the id and the superego?

Defense mechanisms

What type of thinking is primary process?

It is associated with pleasure and instincts. This process does not involve logic or time.

Which part of the mind is controlled by *primary process* thinking?

The id. The id is not influenced by reality and focuses on pleasure and instinct (primary processes).

What is psychotherapy?

A treatment technique. This treatment ranges from strengthening useful ego defenses (in supportive therapy) to challenging detrimental ego defenses and uncovering unconscious conflicts (in expressive therapy), improving self-esteem, and improving relationships.

What is the purpose of psychotherapy?

To improve functionality. It helps to support defenses and functioning, reduce anxiety/stress, help relaxation, work on a specific conflict, improve coping skills, have healthier relationships, more enjoyment/fulfillment in life, and so forth.

What are the differences between psychodynamic psychotherapy and psychoanalysis?

1. Time
   a. Psychoanalysis: 1 hour, 3 to 5× per week for 3 to 4 years
   b. Psychotherapy: 1 hour, 1 to 2× per week for 2 to 20 years
2. Level of therapist's participation:
   a. Psychoanalysis: The therapist mainly listens to the patient who lies on the couch and helps *steer* the patient, clarify, question, gently confront, encourage, interpret, analyze, and so forth.
   b. Psychotherapy: The therapist is more interactive while both he or she and the patient sit in chairs facing each other.

What are the three main techniques used in psychoanalysis and psychodynamic psychotherapy to uncover the unconscious?

Free association, dream interpretations, and transference interpretations

Which technique is used to describe the patient expressing "whatever comes to mind?"	Free association
How does the unconscious mind manifest impulses, wishes, and fears?	Through dreams, slips of the tongue, and forgetting significant things
What is the purpose of a defense mechanism?	*Maintaining the ego* or decreasing anxiety and maintaining a sense of self
What are the mature defense mechanisms?	Humor Altruism Sublimation Suppression
What are the immature defense mechanisms?	Acting out Denial Displacement Dissociation Fixation Identification Isolation Projection Rationalization Reaction formation Regression Repression Splitting
Which defense mechanism causes a patient to take his uncomfortable feelings toward an unacceptable target and aim it at a more acceptable target?	Displacement
Which defense mechanism allows one to use a socially acceptable way to combat an unacceptable impulse?	Sublimation
How does sublimation differ from displacement?	In displacement, the object or person receiving the negative attention is "more tolerable" to the individual (kick dog instead of boss), while in sublimation, the negative attention is channeled into an activity that is socially acceptable (vigorous exercise to relieve stress caused by boss).

Which defense mechanism allows one to find amusement in an otherwise difficult situation?

Humor

If a patient uses intellectualization and isolation of affect as ways to deal with their discomfort, what personality disorder might he have?

Obsessive-compulsive personality disorder (OCPD)

What defense mechanisms are highly associated with OCPD?

Intellectualization (focus on facts about painful things instead of the painful things)

Rationalization (making excuses that seem like a reasonable explanation—e.g., I failed out of medical school because I didn't really like biology anyway.)

Isolation of affect (e.g., I refuse to have emotions about this topic because emotions are too difficult.)

Reaction formation (e.g., I can't deal with the fact that I hate you so I'll give you a gift instead.)

How does rationalization differ from intellectualization?

Rationalization occurs when a person uses excuses to explain an uncomfortable feeling related to an event or person. Intellectualization is when a person defers to factual information in order to deal with or understand uncomfortable feelings.

Which immature defense is used extensively by patients with borderline personality disorder who cannot integrate the good and bad aspects of the same person?

Splitting

Which defense mechanism leads a patient to deal with an uncomfortable situation by "placing it on the back burner?"

Suppression

How does repression differ from suppression?

Repression is an immature defense mechanism that occurs when the unconscious causes us to "forget" painful information while suppression is a mature defense mechanism that allows us to consciously put off painful information and "deal with it later" in order to maintain our composure.

Which defense mechanism is associated with a person dealing with stressful situations in a childlike manner?

Regression

In which personality disorder is repression, regression, and somatization used the most?

Histrionic

Which defense mechanism allows us to place our bad feelings about ourselves onto others?

Projection

How does displacement differ from projection?

Displacement allows us to place our negative emotion about someone else onto another target, while projection allows us to place our negative emotions about ourselves onto another target.

Which defense mechanism causes us to take on the positive and negative behaviors of others?

Identification

Which personality disorders use projection and denial as their primary defense mechanisms?

Paranoid personality disorder

Schizotypal personality disorder

Antisocial personality disorder

Borderline personality disorder

How does denial differ from splitting?

In denial, patients ignore all the bad aspects about something entirely (Bob's dog died but he is still feeding him every night). This is not a conscious action. With splitting, patients cannot see the positive and the negative at the same time (their doctors are either "horrible" or "wonderful" but never "so-so").

If a man "forgets" to return calls to all of the clients he dislikes today, which defense mechanism is at work?

Avoidance

Which two personality disorders primarily utilize avoidance?

Avoidant and dependent personality disorders

If a man who recently embezzled money donates funds to a homeless shelter, what defense mechanism is he using?

Altruism—assisting others to avoid feeling bad about oneself

Which defense mechanism causes an individual to express unacceptable thoughts and feelings in a socially inappropriate manner?

Acting out

Which defense mechanism allows one to avoid a painful situation by acting as if it never happened?

Denial

Which defense mechanism is associated with multiple personalities in which people use cognition to deviate from a part of their personality?

Dissociation

What is the emotional reaction a patient has to his or her physician?

Transference. It occurs when patients unconsciously reexperience relationships in their past during the therapy. This can occur in any relationship (not just with therapists). It can be a useful tool in therapy.

What is the emotional reaction a physician has to a patient?

Countertransference. It has two parts:

(1) Feelings the physician has toward the patient that is related to his or her own past (like transference).

(2) Feelings that a physician has toward the patient that demonstrates how the patient causes most people to feel (patient specific).

What are the merits of recognizing countertransference?

The physician's countertransference can influence the medical treatment of the patient. (A patient is discharged from the hospital without adequate treatment because he yells at his physicians.)

CHAPTER 5

Learning Theory

What is learning theory?

The idea that behavior is learned.

What is behaviorism?

It is a learning theory based on the idea that behavior is a product of learning through association or reinforcement, and thus can be unlearned.

ASSOCIATIVE LEARNING VS. NONASSOCIATIVE LEARNING

What is associative learning?

Learning that occurs when a connection or pairing is made between a particular stimulus and a particular response.

What are associative learning processes?

Classical conditioning

Operant conditioning

What is nonassociative learning?

Nonassociative learning describes behavior change as a result of presentation of one stimulus repeatedly. It also describes learning which has no association with an end stimulus (such as a reward or punishment).

What are nonassociative learning processes?

Observational learning

Habituation

Sensitization

Associative Learning

Classical Conditioning

What is classical conditioning?

Classical conditioning is a way of pairing a stimulus and response. As demonstrated by Pavlov, a novel stimulus (a ringing bell) can be paired with an unconditioned stimulus (food) to elicit an unconditioned or natural response (salivation).

Thus, if a bell (novel stimulus) is rung every time food (unconditioned stimulus) is presented to the dog, it will be *conditioned* to associate the bell with food and will learn to salivate (natural response) at the sound of the bell. This is the conditioned response.

What is the term for the circumstance in which a novel stimulus can elicit a conditioned response?

Stimulus generalization

What is a medical example of classical conditioning?

Phobias are believed to be results of classical conditioning. For example, Mary had a frightening experience on a ship. She may *generalize* that fear so that even the sight of a ship causes her anxiety.

Table 5.1 Pavlov's Classical Conditioning

Stimulus	Natural Response (Unconditioned)	Conditioned Response
Food (odor or sight) (unconditioned stimulus)	Salivation	
Bell (conditioned stimulus)		Salivation

Table 5.2 Medical Example of Classical Conditioning

Stimulus	Natural Response (Unconditioned)	Conditioned Response
Being on a ship (unconditioned stimulus)	Anxiety/fear	
Seeing a ship (conditioned stimulus)		Anxiety/fear

What is extinction?

It is the disappearance of the conditioned response if the conditioned and unconditioned stimuli are never paired again.

Is it possible for the conditioned response to be paired with the conditioned stimulus after extinction has taken place?

Yes, this is called spontaneous recovery.

LEARNED HELPLESSNESS

What does learned helplessness mean?

The effect of repeatedly pairing an adverse stimulus to the inability to escape defines learned helplessness.

What mood disorder may be explained by the theory of learned helplessness?

It has been thought that this theory may explain depression in humans. In this theory, a person has tried repeatedly but unsuccessfully to control external events. The person then pairs any adverse event to the inability to do anything about them. The person then becomes hopeless, depressed, and apathetic.

Imprinting

What is imprinting?

Imprinting describes *phase-sensitive* learning, which occurs most commonly during a very early developmental stage or period of life. During this time, the animal or person imitates the behavior of another stimulus. This learning is rapid and seems to be unrelated to the consequences of the behavior learned.

What is an example of imprinting?

An example of imprinting is when birds follow the first thing they see moving after they hatch. The critical time period is the few moments after birth and the association is made so quickly that the first object that they see suitably moving is what they will follow.

Operant Conditioning

What is operant conditioning?

It is the idea that a behavior is learned because of the reward or punishment associated with it.

What are the different kinds of operant conditioning?

Positive reinforcement

Negative reinforcement

Punishment

Extinction

What are reinforcers?

Any event or stimulus that increases the likelihood of the behavior occurring again

What is positive reinforcement?

Presentation of a rewarding stimulus after a certain behavior is performed. For example, parents may reward their children with ice cream (positive reinforcer) when their rooms are clean, thus increasing the likelihood that the children will clean their rooms.

What is negative reinforcement?

Removal of an aversive stimulus after a certain behavior is performed. For example, parents may exempt the children that clean their rooms from having to take out the trash, thus increasing the likelihood that the children will clean their rooms.

What type of reinforcement increases the likelihood of a behavior occurring again?

Positive and negative reinforcement

What is shaping?

Shaping is learning that occurs when a person is rewarded for a behavior which is similar to a desired behavior. Subsequently, only behavior which is more and more similar to the particular desired behavior is rewarded.

When is shaping used?

It is a progressive modification of behavior which occurs by reinforcement of behavior which is close to the desired outcome.

What is the definition of punishment?

Presentation of an aversive stimulus to *reduce* the likelihood of an unwanted behavior occurring.

What is the definition of extinction in operant conditioning?

Extinction is the disappearance of a certain behavior when the reinforcement is no longer present.

What is an example of extinction?

A rat that is initially trained to press a bar if rewarded with food will quickly cease to press the bar if food is no longer obtained by the behavior.

What are the different schedules of reinforcement?

There are five types of reinforcement schedules:

Continuous—every time behavior is performed

Fixed ratio—set number of times

Variable ratio—random number of times

Fixed interval—set amount of time

Variable interval—random amount of time

Which reinforcement shows the fastest extinction when reinforcement is taken away?

Continuous

What is variable ratio reinforcement?

Reinforcement is given at a variable time interval after the behavior is performed. This type of reinforcement shows the slowest extinction when the reinforcement is taken away. Slot machines are an example of variable ratio reinforcement.

What is the difference between classical and operant conditioning?

Classical conditioning refers to behaviors *learned by association* of stimuli and responses whereas *operant conditioning* refers to behaviors *learned by the reward and reinforcement* associated with them.

NONASSOCIATIVE LEARNING

What is observational learning?

In observational learning, the observer's behaviors change based upon observing the model's behaviors. The consequences of the model's behaviors, whether they are positive or negative, have an effect on the observer's behaviors.

If a person observes others and then imitates their behavior, what is that behavior called?

Modeling. Modeling is a type of observational learning. Compared to operant learning it is a more efficient and faster type of learning. Modeling is useful in acquiring new skills.

What four aspects are needed in order for a person to be able to model?

Attention to the model

Retention of details

Motor reproduction

Motivation and opportunity

Where in medicine is modeling used?

The common saying, "see one, do one, teach one," is a description of modeling in learning how to do medical procedures.

Can modeling have a negative outcome?

Yes. Modeling may occur when a child models the actions of a parent with a particular phobia and hence also acquires the same phobia or perpetuation of abuse by an abused person.

Can modeling have a positive outcome?

Yes. Modeling may involve *other* types of learning, e.g., seeing a role model/mentor's behavior achieve a positive result would then act as a positive reinforcer (which would be an example of *operant conditioning*).

What is habituation?

Habituation occurs when stimulus presentation results in decreased responsiveness.

What is an example of habituation?

You may notice the hum of the air conditioner when it first comes on, but due to habituation, your awareness of that continual hum will decrease and you can focus on your studies.

How is habituation used in medicine?

Habituation is used to overcome phobias. Some of the specific techniques using habituation are flooding and systemic desensitization.

How do you describe flooding?

It is excessive presentation of the stimulus to achieve quick habituation by preventing escape and forcing a reduction in the associated behavior.

What is an example of flooding?

One could force an individual with an obsession about germs to touch a toilet.

How do you describe systematic desensitization?

In systematic desensitization, the patient is *gradually* exposed to anxiety-producing situations while simultaneously teaching relaxation or anxiety-reducing techniques.

What is sensitization?

Sensitization occurs when stimulus presentation results in *increased* responsiveness and/or generalization of response to other stimuli.

What is an example of sensitization?

Joe is alone in a dark house when he hears a sudden loud noise. He suddenly becomes more aware of every little sound in the house.

CHAPTER 6

Substance Abuse Issues

What is drug addiction?

It implies drug dependence in which the drug seeking behavior has taken over a major part of the individual's life.

What is drug abuse?

If a person takes a drug that produces harmful effects on the individual without meeting the criteria for dependence.

How is drug dependence defined in the Diagnostic and Statistical Manual of Mental Disorders—Fourth Edition (DSM-IV)?

Maladaptive pattern of substance use leading to clinically significant impairment or distress which may or may not have physiologic dependence.

How is physiologic dependence defined?

The presence of tolerance and/or a specific drug withdrawal syndrome.

What pathway is involved in the chemical rewards of drug use?

Stimulation of the *dopaminergic pathway* from the *ventral tegmental area* (VTA) to the *nucleus accumbens*.

How do cocaine and amphetamines cause rewards through this pathway?

Cocaine and amphetamines exert their effects by increasing dopamine release and decreasing its reuptake.

How do opiates cause rewards through this pathway?

Opiates exert their effects by the release of opioid peptides that stimulate neurons along this pathway.

How does alcohol cause rewards through this pathway?

Alcohol exerts its effects by increasing the release of both γ-aminobutyric acid (GABA) and opioid peptides.

How does nicotine cause rewards through this pathway?

Nicotine works by increasing acetylcholine release.

What factors affect how quickly and to what magnitude the chemical rewards are felt after ingestion of a drug?

1. Route of administration: The faster through the blood-brain barrier, the greater the euphoria and higher likelihood of addiction (e.g., IV > smoking > oral [pills])
2. Chemical composition of the drug (increasing purity → increased and faster effects)
3. Genetic differences between people (relates to receptor stimulation)
4. Associated stimuli (i.e., drug paraphernalia, other conditional stimuli)

What is the Himmelsbach hypothesis?

The Himmelsbach hypothesis is a theory on drug dependence/drug use rewards that states that drug dependence is a cyclic process in which the patient goes from a drug-free state to one in which the drug effects are being experienced in a positive manner. The patient then develops tolerance to the drug effects in the form of neuroadaptation which then progresses to a withdrawal syndrome. This withdrawal is followed by recovery from the neuroadaptive state and entry into a drug-free state.

What are the three important observations that Himmelsbach made?

1. There is a common association between tolerance and a specific withdrawal syndrome.
2. The nature of the withdrawal syndrome is opposite to the acute effects of the drug.
3. The withdrawal syndrome is most intense when the drug leaves the brain rapidly.

What are some characteristics of drug withdrawal?

Anxiety

Autonomic signs (elevated heart rate, elevated blood pressure)

Increased gastrointestinal (GI) motility leading to diarrhea

Other specific symptoms

What are the four central tenets that must be addressed in order to successfully treat drug dependence?

1. The positive reinforcements/reward effects of the drug must be reduced.
2. The negative reinforcements (withdrawal symptoms) must be treated, either by giving a substitute drug or by symptomatically treating the effects of drug removal.
3. Detoxification—complete removal of the drug of dependence from the patient's system.
4. Relapse into drug use may be preventable by reducing the desire for the drug or by reducing cravings for the drug.

How should withdrawal symptoms be prevented/treated during detoxification?

Withdrawal symptoms may be prevented/treated by administering a substitute drug that cause cross-dependence by suppressing the withdrawal symptoms from another drug, or by symptomatically treating the effects of drug removal.

How can the positive reinforcement effects of drugs be reduced?

1. Giving specific receptor antagonists to prevent the binding of receptors by the drug of dependence; therefore, precipitating withdrawal and preventing the effects of the drug (e.g., naloxone or naltrexone treatment for opiates).
2. Giving receptor inverse agonists that cause adverse effects when the drug is consumed (e.g., sarmazenil for alcohol dependence).
3. Giving antibodies for the drug that prevent the drug from reaching the brain; thereby, preventing the pleasant effects of the drug by destroying it before the drug gets to its target (have been shown beneficial in cocaine and nicotine dependence).
4. Converting reward to punishment (e.g., the use of disulfiram or Antabuse, for alcohol dependence).

5. Giving dopamine or opiate antagonists to cause general inhibition of the reward pathways.
6. Negative discriminative stimuli (e.g., telling the patients that their drug of choice will be ineffective; therefore, they stay away from it).
   Note: Points 2 and 3 are still experimental.

How does disulfiram work?

Disulfiram inhibits aldehyde dehydrogenase in the liver, so that when combined with alcohol, it cannot be fully metabolized leading to flushing, headache, and nausea.

What side effect of opiate antagonists may result in compliance problems?

Anhedonia

What are the three major ways of reducing negative reinforcement/ withdrawal?

1. Substitute drugs that act as agonists for the same receptor, and therefore, prevent severe withdrawal (i.e., using methadone to treat heroin or opiate dependence).
2. Substitution by partial agonist for the same receptor, thereby, preventing severe withdrawal and counteracting the effects of the drug if it is taken.
3. Substitution of a different route of administration to prevent some of the adverse effects of the drug itself while still preventing withdrawal (i.e., using the nicotine patch for smoking cessation).

What criteria should be used when selecting a substitute drug for treating negative reinforcement?

Substitute drugs should be:

Less rewarding

Less damaging

More manageable

Provide less positive reinforcement

What are the major problems with using positive and negative reinforcement treatments?

To use positive reinforcement treatments, the patient must undergo detoxification first.

Negative reinforcement treatments may lead to polydrug abuse, especially if substitution methods are used.

What is the basic principle behind detoxification?

Detoxification uses the principle of substitution with a drug of cross-dependence or different route of administration to allow for safer, slower withdrawal from the drug of dependence. It should not be used to precipitate withdrawal.

What percentage of patients who become drug free relapse?

75%, most within the first year

What are the most common factors that precipitate relapse?

Peer pressure

Boredom

Cravings

Reinstatement of a positively reinforcing lifestyle

What modalities have been associated with decreased incidence of relapse?

Joining self-help groups → providing a different type of peer pressure and reinforcement

Cognitive therapy → helps develop new and different coping skills

What is the most likely reason for relapse?

Cravings are the most common reason for relapse. Cravings are caused by memories of the positive rewards of drug use or by conditioning cues that are endogenous or exogenous.

How can cravings be treated to prevent relapse?

Cravings may be treated by reducing the desire for the drug, providing a substitute for the drug reward, reducing endogenous cues for cravings (i.e., by using anxiolytics or antidepressants), reducing the conditional anticipation of the reward (i.e., giving naltrexone to an alcoholic), or by reducing pseudowithdrawal symptoms.

What are some of the medical effects of drug abuse?

Increased risk of lung disease and cancer (with smoking)

Increased risk of human immunodeficiency virus (HIV), hepatitis, and other infections with intravenous (IV) drug use

Acute and chronic toxicities

What are some of the nonmedical consequences of drug abuse?	Sociological problems such as violence, crime, and poverty Acute impairment leading to reduced cognition or restraint Other risky behaviors (e.g., increased likelihood of sexual violence)
What are the acute symptoms of ethanol toxicity?	Vomiting (with risk of possible aspiration due to decreased mental status) Respiratory depression Coma Death
What are the chronic symptoms of ethanol toxicity?	Psychiatric symptoms (depression, hallucinations) Neurological signs (dementia, vascular problems, and neuropathies) GI tract malfunction (cirrhosis of the liver, pancreatitis, and GI cancer) Cardiovascular disease (cardiomyopathy, hypertension)
What are the clinical manifestations of fetal alcohol syndrome?	Pre- and postnatal retardation of growth and cognition Distinct craniofacial abnormalities Central nervous system (CNS) damage Attention deficits Low intelligence quotient (IQ)
What are the acute and chronic medical effects of tobacco use?	Acute: Nausea, vomiting, initial autonomic stimulation followed by autonomic block Chronic: Diseases of the lungs (cancer, bronchitis, emphysema, asthma, and so forth) Diseases of the cardiovascular system (arteriosclerosis, atheroma, hypertension, coronary thrombosis, and so forth) Diseases of the CNS (stroke, neurodegenerative disease) Fetal growth retardation in pregnant women

What is the most common form of drug dependence?	Caffeine dependence, which is seen in 60% to 70% of the population
What are the effects of caffeine?	Caffeinism: Anxiety, insomnia, palpitations, and gastric irritation Cardiovascular system conditions: Hypertension and cardiac dysrhythmias, possibly a role in coronary thrombosis
What is the mechanism of action of cocaine?	Cocaine is a stimulant that works by preventing the reuptake of catecholamine transmitters, such as dopamine and norepinephrine, in the brain and autonomic nervous system.
What are the physiologic effects of cocaine use?	Vasoconstriction Tachycardia Hyperthermia Hypertension Cardiac dysrhythmias Stroke Paranoid psychosis (in chronic use)
What is the most likely mechanism of paranoid psychosis in chronic cocaine users?	Dopamine potentiation
What is the mechanism of action of amphetamines?	Amphetamines are stimulants that work by reducing the reuptake and cause the release of stored amine transmitters such as dopamine, norepinephrine, and serotonin.
What are the acute and chronic effects of amphetamine use?	Vasoconstriction Tachycardia Hyperthermia Hypertension Cardiac dysrhythmias Stroke Paranoid psychosis Neurotoxicity
What is the mechanism of action of dissociative anesthetic drugs like ketamine and phencyclidine?	Dissociative anesthetics work by blocking *n*-methyl-D-aspartate (NMDA) receptors and sigma receptors in the CNS.

What are the effects of dissociative anesthetic use?	Amnesia Confusion Paranoid delusions Hallucinations Violent behavior Hyperthermia
What is the mechanism of action of marijuana?	Marijuana is a tetrahydrocannabinoid that works on cannabinoid receptors, a member of G protein-linked receptors. These affect monoamine and GABA neurons in the basal ganglia, hippocampus, and cerebellum.
What are the chronic toxicities associated with marijuana use?	Lung cancer Poor memory and motivation Flashbacks Testosterone suppression Immunosuppression Fetal damage
Where are the opioid receptors located in the brain and what is the function of each receptor?	Periaqueductal grey matter → responsible for analgesia Area postrema → responsible for nausea and vomiting Ventral medulla → responsible for respiratory depression Edinger-Westphal nucleus → responsible for the pinpoint pupil response (due to extreme miosis) Nucleus accumbens → responsible for euphoria
What are the three types of opioid receptors?	Mu Kappa Delta
What peptide transmitters work at opioid receptor and which receptors do they act on?	Enkephalins act on mu and delta receptors, main actions are at delta receptors Beta-endorphins act on mu and delta receptors equally Dynorphins act on kappa receptors

Describe the mechanism of action of opioids at their receptors.

Opioid receptors are G protein-coupled receptors with seven membrane spanning segments. Activation of the receptors causes changes in cyclic adenosine monophosphate (cAMP), Ca^{2+}, and so forth, leading to inhibition of neuronal excitation.

How do strong agonists cause the effects of opioids?

Strong agonists have high affinity for the receptor and high efficacy to produce a conformational change that activates the receptor.

How do antagonists work?

Antagonists have high affinity for the receptor and no efficacy to produce conformational changes that activate the receptor.

What is the difference between strong and partial agonists?

Both strong and partial agonists have high affinity for the receptor; but unlike strong agonists, partial agonists have low efficacy to produce a conformational change that activates the receptor resulting in weak activation of the receptor and antagonization/blockade of the effects of a strong agonist.

What is the difference between opiates and opioids?

Opiates are derived from the opium poppy, while opioids are synthetic or semisynthetic derivatives of drugs derived from the opium poppy.

How do kappa and mu receptors differ?

The difference between kappa receptors and mu receptors is that activation of kappa receptors produces less analgesia (ceiling effect), less respiratory depression/asphyxia (floor effect), and the lack of ability to produce euphoria (less abuse potential).

Which narcotics are strong mu receptor agonists?

Morphine

Fentanyl

Etorphine

Heroin

Hydromorphone

Hydrocodone

	Oxycodone Codeine Meperidine
Which narcotics are partial mu receptor agonists?	Buprenorphine Pentazocine
Which narcotics are moderate/strong or selective kappa receptor agonists?	Nalorphine (moderate) Pentazocine (moderate) Etorphine (strong) Butorphanol (selective) Meperidine (moderate)
Which narcotic is a weak kappa receptor agonist?	Morphine
Which narcotic is a strong delta receptor agonist?	Etorphine
What opioid receptor does the cough suppressant dextromethorphan act upon?	Sigma receptors
Which narcotics are mu receptor antagonists?	Nalorphine Naltrexone (nonnarcotic)
Which narcotics are kappa receptor antagonists?	Buprenorphine Naltrexone (nonnarcotic)
What drug can be used as a narcotic reversal agent?	Naltrexone/Naloxone (aka Narcan)
Which narcotics are metabolized by CYP2D6?	Oxycodone Codeine
What is the significance of being metabolized by CYP2D6?	In drugs that are metabolized by CYP2D6, the active metabolite is morphine.
Which narcotic can be used as an antidiarrheal agent?	Loperamide, which works by reducing GI tract motility.
What is the clinical indication for methadone?	Methadone is used to treat withdrawal from heroin while acting to decrease cravings and risk from associated lifestyle (legal, HIV, hepatitis, and so forth).
What are the symptoms of narcotic overdose?	In narcotic overdoses, CO_2 drive is reduced resulting in respiratory depression and cyanosis and diminished mental status/coma.

What is the route of absorption of ethanol in the body?

The very low molecular weight as well as its water and lipid solubility allow for rapid absorption of ethanol from the GI tract and entry into the brain.

What is the limiting factor in ethanol absorption?

Absorption of ethanol is limited only by the surface area of the stomach.

What is the effect of ethanol's water solubility?

Its water solubility allows absorbed ethanol to be distributed throughout the body water.

What is the mechanism of action of ethanol?

Ethanol's mechanism of action involves entry into the neuronal membrane and disruption of the function of multisubunit proteins such as γ-aminobutryic acid type A ($GABA_A$) receptors, glutamate receptors, and other receptors that conduct ions across the neuronal membrane.

What is the physiologic effect of ethanol's action on GABA receptors?

GABA is the major inhibitory transmitter in the brain, and ethanol potentiation of GABA causes anxiolysis and possibly the reward effects by increasing dopamine release from the nucleus accumbens.

What is the physiologic effect of ethanol's action on glutamate receptors?

Glutamate is a major excitatory transmitter in the brain, and ethanol inhibits glutamate causing amnesia and anesthetic effects and possibly reward effects.

What are the clinically observed effects of ethanol?

Anxiolysis/euphoriant effects

Relaxation

Stress relief

Excitement → aggression and violence

Creativity

Hilarity

Mood elevation

Reduced inhibitions → lack of restraint, sexual behavior/attacks, crime

Anesthetic effects → motor incoordination, loss of balance, slowed reflexes, and rousable loss of consciousness

Coma and death with extremely elevated blood alcohol

How many drinks are needed for a man to reach the legal limit (0.08% blood alcohol content [BAC])?

For a man approximately five drinks = a BAC of 0.1% (above the legal limit)

How many drinks are needed for a woman to reach the legal limit (0.08% BAC)?

For a woman, approximately three drinks = a BAC of 0.105% (above the legal limit)

How is ethanol eliminated from the body?

Ethanol is eliminated unchanged through the breath, sweat, and urine. Ninety-five percent of the ethanol ingested is metabolized in the liver.

How is ethanol metabolized in the liver?

Alcohol metabolism is a zero-order process in which alcohol is converted by alcohol dehydrogenase to aldehydes, and then the aldehydes are converted by aldehyde dehydrogenase to acetate.

What is zero-order elimination of a drug?

Zero-order elimination occurs when a constant amount of drug is eliminated from the body per unit of time.

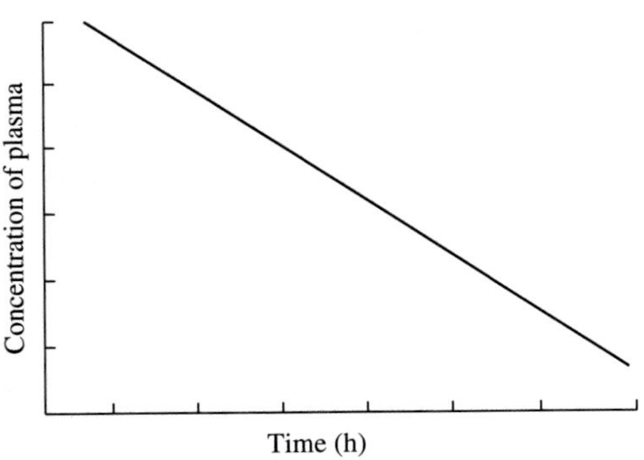

Figure 6.1 Zero-Order Elimination. (*Note:* Drugs have a constant elimination. A constant amount of drug is eliminated per unit time.)

What is the limiting factor in ethanol metabolism by the liver?

The limiting factor in alcohol metabolism is the availability of nicotinamide adenine dinucleotide (NAD) and nicotinamide adenine dinucleotide plus hydrogen (NADH), which is used by aldehyde dehydrogenase.

Which metabolic process is responsible for the toxic effects of alcohol?

The toxic effects of alcohol are related to metabolism of alcohol to aldehydes, the build up of which causes liver and tissue damage, flushing, nausea, and headache.

What are the chronic effects of alcohol ingestion?

Development of tolerance

Psychological dependence

Physiologic dependence (this includes tolerance and withdrawal)

Medical problems

What are the three types of tolerance?

Metabolic tolerance—allows for more rapid metabolism and excretion

Behavioral tolerance—involves learning to perform a task while intoxicated as if the person is not intoxicated

Neuroadaptation—involves the evolution of alterations in the brain that help to overcome the effects of the drug

What are the elements of neuroadaptation theory?

Neuroadaptation theory describes the development of physiologic dependence by initial alterations of brain neurochemistry with acute drug use that is followed by the development of tolerance to the drug's effects with chronic use. This tolerance and the presence of a withdrawal syndrome after rapid removal of the drug exposes this neuroadaptation. In the absence of the drug, the brain will readapt to its predrug use state.

What are the acute symptoms of alcohol withdrawal?

Acute alcohol withdrawal results in a hangover, with symptoms including anxiety, dysphoria, photophobia, tremors/shakes, sleep disturbance/decreased rapid eye movement (REM) sleep, vivid nightmares, monoclinic jerks, and formication.

What are symptoms of withdrawal from chronic alcohol use?

Minor signs include anxiety, dysphoria, depression, and sleep disturbance.

Major signs include delirium/confusion, terror, hallucinations, severe tremor, seizures, and autonomic signs.

How is alcohol withdrawal treated?

Benzodiazepines, such as diazepam for suppression of withdrawal symptoms (reduces them down to only a tremor)

Vitamins (particularly thiamine) to treat underlying vitamin deficiencies seen in long-term alcoholism

Antihypertensives to suppress underlying hypertension that can be made worse by the physiologic withdrawal process

What is the relapse rate in the first year after alcohol detoxification?

75%

What are the most common reasons for relapse in alcoholics?

Memories/conditioning

Peer pressure

Genetics

Rapid reinstatement of physiologic dependence

What types of treatment can be used to prevent relapse in alcoholics?

Self-help groups

Psychological treatment

Pharmacotherapy (naltrexone, disulfiram, or acamprosate)

CHAPTER 7

Analyzing Sleep: Normal and Sleep Disorders

NORMAL SLEEP

What are the normal stages of sleep?

REM (rapid eye movement) and NREM (nonrapid eye movement).

NREM is divided into four stages: 1, 2, 3, and 4.

What is slow wave sleep?

Slow wave sleep occurs during stages 3 and 4 of NREM sleep. It is also known as *delta sleep* and is the deepest, relaxed portion of sleep. Electroencephalogram (EEG) shows delta waves, which are the lowest frequency waves.

What waveforms are seen in REM sleep?

Beta waves. These are of highest frequency.

Where else are beta waves seen?

They are found over the frontal lobes in a person who is awake with his or her eyes open. These are associated with a person who is alert and actively concentrating (You!). In a person who is awake with his or her eyes closed, alpha waves are seen typically over the occipital and posterior parietal lobes.

What waveforms are associated with Stages 1 and 2 of NREM?

Stage 1 (light sleep) is associated with theta waves and Stage 2 (deeper sleep) is associated with sleep spindles and K-complexes.

On average, how much time does a normal adult spend in each stage of sleep?

REM—25%

NREM—75%

Within NREM sleep:

Stage 1—5%

Stage 2—45%

Stages 3 and 4—25%

What is REM latency?

REM latency is the length of time after falling asleep before REM sleep occurs.

What is the length of REM latency in an adult?

REM latency in an adult is approximately 90 minutes. The REM sleep cycle then repeats itself approximately every 90 minutes thereafter.

Besides, rapid eye movements, what other physiologic changes occur in REM sleep?

Pulse, respiration, blood pressure, and brain oxygen use increase. There is penile/clitoral erection, dreaming, and decreased skeletal muscle tone.

How is this different from the physiologic changes in NREM sleep?

In NREM, blood pressure, pulse, and respiration slow. There may also be intermittent limb movements.

Tip: This makes sense—if your blood pressure (BP) and pulse are up and your genitals are aroused, NREM sleep wouldn't be very restful!

Which neurotransmitter usually initiates sleep?

Serotonin. It is released from the dorsal raphe nucleus and is a derivative of tryptophan. It increases total sleep time and slow wave activity.

Tip: Turkey is high in tryptophan—this is why you get sleepy after a big Thanksgiving dinner.

Which neurotransmitters are involved in REM sleep?

Acetylcholine (ACh) from the basal forebrain and norepinephrine (NE) from the locus ceruleus. ACh increases REM sleep and NE decreases it.

How does REM change with age?

Time spent in REM decreases with age.

What effect does dopamine have on the sleep cycle?

Dopamine increases wakefulness. Thus, antipsychotics, which block dopamine, can result in increased sedation. Stimulants, which increase both NE and dopamine, promote wakefulness.

ABNORMAL SLEEP

Approximately how many adults experience sleep disorders every year?

About one in three

What is the most common type of sleep disorder?

Insomnia, which includes problems initiating and maintaining sleep.

What is a primary sleep disorder?

Sleep disturbances that arise from endogenous sources, not from substance use, medical problems, or other psychiatric problems. Primary sleep disorders are divided into two major categories:

1. Parasomnias
2. Dyssomnias

What is the difference between dyssomnias and parasomnias?

Dyssomnias are due to dysfunctional sleep regulation characterized by problems initiating or maintaining sleep, or excessive daytime sleepiness.

Parasomnias involve abnormal behaviors or physiologic events during sleep, rather than abnormal functioning of the usual mechanisms of sleep. These include sleep terror disorder, sleepwalking disorder, and nightmare disorder.

Name the five major dyssomnias

1. Primary insomnia
2. Primary hypersomnia
3. Narcolepsy
4. Breathing related sleep disorder
5. Circadian rhythm sleep disorder

How long must you have problems with insomnia before primary insomnia can be diagnosed?

At least a month

What interventions other than medications can be useful in insomnia?

Set a regular bedtime, abstain from caffeine and alcohol, use the bed only for sleep and sex, and avoid daytime naps and strenuous exercise or large meals just before bedtime. Collectively, this is referred to as *sleep hygiene.*

What is the subtype of recurrent primary hypersomnia associated with obesity, impulsivity, hyperphagia, hypersexuality, and disorganized thought called?

Kleine-Levin syndrome

Other than daytime sleepiness and "sleep attacks," what symptoms are classically associated with narcolepsy?

1. Cataplexy—sudden loss of muscle tone associated with strong emotions
2. Hypnagogic and hypnopompic hallucinations—REM intrusions that occur during the transition period between sleep and wakefulness. (Hypnagogic occur when going to sleep and hypnopompic occur during waking up.)
3. Sleep paralysis—inability to move just before going to sleep or awakening.

Which class of drugs is normally used to treat narcolepsy?

Stimulants, for example, Ritalin

Why are people with breathing related sleeping disorder chronically sleepy during the day?

During the night they frequently stop breathing and then are awoken by hypoxia. These frequent arousals prevent the patients from getting deep, restful sleep.

What is the most common cause of breathing related sleep disorder and how is it treated?

Obstructive sleep apnea (OSA). Treatment—continuous positive airway pressure (CPAP) and possibly removal of tonsils and adenoids (ideally weight loss would be primary intervention in the obese).

In a patient with excessive fatigue, what might the patients' bed partner tell you about his or her sleep that might lead you to suspect obstructive sleep apnea?

Loud snoring and periods of time where the patient appears to stop breathing

In a person with sleep problems related to OSA, why might you avoid benzodiazepines?

You risk further compromising the patient's ventilation.

What are the three most common causes of a circadian rhythm sleep disorder?

1. Delayed sleep phase—"night owls," more common in adolescents and tends to improve with age
2. Jet lag—typically resolves over several days
3. Shift work—e.g., working the night shift

During which phase of sleep would you expect nightmares to occur in?

REM

What are the similarities between sleep terrors and sleepwalking?

Both are more common in children and may involve semicomplex to complex motor behaviors. Patients tend to be amnestic for both and in adulthood they are equally prevalent in men and women (1% prevalence of sleep terrors and 2% prevalence of sleepwalking). Both occur in slow wave sleep.

How could you clinically differentiate sleep terror from sleepwalking?

Sleep terror has strong component of autonomic arousal and fear, often beginning with a terrified scream, and a lesser element of semipurposeful motor behaviors. Sleepwalking has minimal autonomic arousal/fear and motor behaviors are usually more complex.

What is the treatment of sleep terrors and sleepwalking?

Benzodiazepines. They reduce slow wave sleep, the time at which these parasomnias occur.

OTHER SLEEP CHANGES

What polysomnogram (PSG) findings are characteristic of major depression?

Reduced slow wave sleep (less delta waves), frequent nighttime awakenings, increased sleep latency (time until falling asleep), short REM latency (REM cycle starts sooner than normal 90 minutes onset), and early morning waking.

Tip: Low serotonin is associated with depression; therefore you would expect reduced total sleep and slow wave sleep!

A common feature of Alzheimer's is reduced ACh, given this what PSG changes are seen in an individual with Alzheimer's?

Decreased slow wave and REM sleep

CHAPTER 8

Genetics: Role of Genetics in Human Behavior

GENETIC STUDIES

What type of study uses a family tree to show the occurrence of traits and diseases throughout generations?	Pedigree study
What type of study compares the frequency of disease in a proband (affected individual) with its frequency in the general population?	Family risk study
What type of study compares monozygotic and dizygotic twins to determine the effects of genetic factors from environmental factors of disease?	Adoption study
This term describes if both twins have a given trait.	Concordance
What type of twins is more likely to have a higher likelihood of having a disease that is genetic in origin?	Monozygotic twins

PSYCHIATRIC DISORDERS AND THEIR GENETIC ORIGINS

What is the prevalence of schizophrenia in the general population?	1%
In which gender is schizophrenia more likely?	Equal in males and females

Which persons have a higher likelihood of developing schizophrenia?	Persons with a close genetic relationship
Genetic markers on which chromosome(s) are associated with schizophrenia?	1, 6, 8, and 13
What is the likelihood of developing schizophrenia if you are a first-degree relative of a proband?	10%
What is the likelihood of developing schizophrenia if someone is a child with both parents who have the disorder?	40%
What is the likelihood of developing schizophrenia if you are the monozygotic twin of a person with the disorder?	50%
What is the likelihood of developing any mood disorder if you are a first-degree relative of a proband with bipolar disorder?	25%
What is the likelihood of developing any mood disorder if someone is a child with both parents who have bipolar disorder?	60%
What is the likelihood of developing bipolar disorder if you are the monozygotic twin of a person with the disorder?	80% to 90%
Is the genetic component stronger for schizophrenia or bipolar disorder?	Bipolar disorder
In which gender is the lifetime prevalence of a major depressive disorder higher?	Females
What is the percentage of males who will develop a major depressive disorder in their lifetime?	10%
What is the percentage of females who will develop a major depressive disorder in their lifetime?	15% to 20%
Do personality disorders have a higher concordance in monozygotic twins demonstrating that they have a genetic component?	Yes
If a proband has antisocial personality disorder, what psychiatric condition(s) will be prevalent in relatives?	Alcoholism Attention deficit hyperactivity disorder (ADHD)

If a proband has avoidant personality disorder, what psychiatric condition(s) will be prevalent in relatives?	Anxiety disorder
If a proband has borderline personality disorder, what psychiatric condition(s) will be prevalent in relatives?	Major depressive disorder Substance abuse
If a proband has histrionic personality disorder, what psychiatric condition(s) will be prevalent in relatives?	Somatization disorder
If a proband has schizotypal personality disorder, what psychiatric condition(s) will be prevalent in relatives?	Schizophrenia

NEUROPSYCHIATRIC DISORDERS AND THEIR GENETIC BASIS

In which disease is there a diminution of cognitive functioning and a likelihood of genetic influence?	Alzheimer's disease
Which chromosome is defective in Down syndrome and implicated in some cases of Alzheimer's disease?	Chromosome 21
What other chromosome(s) have been identified to be associated with Alzheimer's disease?	Chromosomes 1 and 14
Which gene has been implicated in Alzheimer's disease?	Apolipoprotein E4 (Apo E4)
In which chromosome is the ApoE4 gene located?	Chromosome 19
What disease has an abnormal gene on the short end of chromosome 4?	Huntington's disease
What is the most common genetic cause of mental retardation?	Down syndrome
What is the second most common genetic cause of mental retardation?	Fragile X syndrome
In addition to fragile X, in what other neuropsychiatric condition is there X-linked transmission?	Lesch-Nyhan syndrome
What disorder, characterized by verbal and motor tics, has a genetic component?	Tourette disorder

ALCOHOLISM AND ITS GENETIC BASIS

What is the prevalence of alcoholism in children of alcoholics compared to the general population?	4× more prevalent
What is the concordance rate of alcoholism in monozygotic twins?	60%
What is the concordance rate of alcoholism in dizygotic twins?	30%
Which gender offspring of alcoholics is more likely to become alcoholics themselves?	Male offspring
At which age group is the genetic influence of alcoholism strongest in males?	Males <20 years of age

CHAPTER 9

Pharmacological and Therapeutic Treatments in Psychiatry

What is the only property of benzodiazepines to which tolerance does not develop?

Tolerance does not develop to the antianxiety/anxiolytic effects of benzos; tolerance may develop to the hypnotic, muscle relaxant, and anticonvulsant effects (e.g., benzodiazepines should not be used for long term seizure control).

Which benzodiazepines are considered anxiolytics?

Alprazolam

Chlordiazepoxide

Clonazepam

Clorazepate

Diazepam

Lorazepam

Which benzodiazepines are considered hypnotics (used to facilitate sleep)?

Quazepam

Midazolam

Estazolam

Flurazepam

Temazepam

Triazolam

What drug can be used to reverse the effects of benzodiazepines?

Flumazenil (Romazicon)

What is the general mechanism of action of benzodiazepines?

Benzodiazepines target the γ-aminobutryic acid type A ($GABA_A$) chloride channel receptor resulting in an increase in the receptor's affinity for γ-aminobutyric acid (GABA) and causing the ion channels to *remain open longer* thus allowing more chloride ions to pass through.

Is there a danger in taking benzodiazepines during pregnancy?

Benzodiazepines can cross the placenta, and therefore should not be taken during pregnancy if possible. It may cause cleft palate in fetuses exposed in utero.

How many phases are there in benzodiazepine metabolism?

There are three phases.

Phase 1: The R1 and R2 residues are oxidized.

Phase 2: The R3 residue is hydroxylated.

Phase 3: The hydroxyl compounds are conjugated with glucuronic acid.

Where does benzodiazepine metabolism occur?

In the liver

Which benzodiazepines skip phase 1 and/or phase 2 of metabolism and are therefore safe to give to patients with liver failure?

Desmethyldiazepam

Oxazepam

Temazepam

Lorazepam

Midazolam

Triazolam

What three substances should be avoided by patients taking benzodiazepines?

The drug cimetidine, oral contraceptives, and grapefruit juice (they slow phases 1 and 2 of metabolism). They are known to inhibit cytochrome P450. Additionally, some human immunodeficiency virus (HIV) antivirals, Cipro, and Ketoconazole have been shown to slow benzodiazepine metabolism.

What are the symptoms of benzodiazepine withdrawal?

Anxiety

Insomnia

Irritability
Muscle aches
Weakness
Tremor
Loss of appetite

What are the possible side effects of benzodiazepines?

Drowsiness
Confusion
Motor incoordination
Cognitive impairment
Anterograde amnesia

In what chronic disease state is midazolam contraindicated?

Chronic obstructive pulmonary disease (COPD)—it can exaggerate the effects on respiration resulting in an increased risk of death

Which benzodiazepines are considered to be high potency?

Triazolam
Alprazolam
Clonazepam

Which benzodiazepines are considered to be low potency?

Diazepam
Chlordiazepoxide
Oxazepam

Which benzodiazepine is indicated for treatment of alcohol withdrawal seizures (delirium tremens)?

Chlordiazepoxide
Oxazepam
Diazepam

Which benzodiazepine(s) is indicated for treatment of status epilepticus, as they can be given intravenous (IV)?

Diazepam and lorazepam

Why are benzodiazepines safer pharmacologic agents to use to treat anxiety than barbiturates?

Less potential for abuse
Higher therapeutic index

What is the mechanism of action of barbiturates?

Barbiturates target the $GABA_A$ chloride channel receptor and its action on chloride entry into the cell, which results in membrane hyperpolarization. There is an increase in the duration of the chloride channel opening and a decrease in neuron excitability.

What is the mechanism of action and common use of Buspirone?	It is a 5 hydroxytryptamine receptor 1A (5-HT_{1A}) (serotonin) agonist that may be used to treat anxiety, particularly useful in those for whom benzodiazepine therapy is contraindicated (the elderly and those with a history of substance abuse).
Which short-acting antianxiety agent is used to treat insomnia?	Zolpidem tartrate
What is the most commonly prescribed class of drugs for the treatment of depression?	SSRIs (selective serotonin reuptake inhibitors)
What is the mechanism of action of SSRIs?	They work by inhibiting neuronal uptake of serotonin, thereby increasing the synaptic concentration of serotonin.
What are the names of commonly prescribed SSRIs?	Fluoxetine Fluvoxamine Paroxetine Sertraline Citaprolam
What serious side effects have a greater incidence associated with the SSRI Paroxetine?	Extrapyramidal effects and sexual dysfunction
Which SSRI can be used in children?	None! *All* are now black-boxed with a warning about children and adolescents!
Which SSRIs are now available in generic form (and may be a better choice for patients with a limited budget)?	Fluoxetine (Prozac) Paroxetine Sertraline will be available soon
Why does fluoxetine have a greater association with drug interactions than other SSRIs?	It has the greatest P-450 inhibition of all the SSRIs.
Why is insomnia a troubling side effect of fluoxetine?	It causes the most central nervous system (CNS) activation of the SSRIs.
Which SSRI is most likely to cause gastrointestinal disturbances?	Sertraline (Zoloft)

Which SSRI is currently only indicated for obsessive-compulsive disorder?	Fluvoxamine
What is the drug classification of bupropion (Wellbutrin)?	It is a SNRI (selective norepinephrine reuptake inhibitor)
What is the major indication for bupropion?	Major depressive disorder
What is another common indication for bupropion?	Smoking cessation
What is a problematic side effect of the antidepressant trazodone seen mostly in males?	Priapism
What is the mechanism of action of tricyclic antidepressants?	Tricyclic antidepressants inhibit the neuronal reuptake of both serotonin and norepinephrine; thus, increasing the availability of serotonin and norepinephrine at the synaptic cleft.
What are the names of commonly prescribed tricyclic antidepressants?	Amitriptyline Clomipramine Doxepin Desipramine Imipramine Nortriptyline
What is a troubling side effect of tricyclic antidepressants and a key sign indicating overdose or intoxication?	Tricyclic antidepressants have anticholinergic effects including dry mouth, blurry vision, constipation, urinary retention, confusion, and memory deficits. Clinical correlate: The combination of dry mouth, blurry vision, and confusion may be a clue to tricyclic overdose or ingestion in some cases, especially if it is known that tricyclics were available to the patient. Other signs of overdose or ingestion include prolonged QT interval, atrioventricular (AV) node block, and orthostatic hypotension.
What is a common indication for prescribing tricyclic antidepressants?	Refractory depression that has failed other classes of antidepressants. In addition, prior response, good tolerability, and/or patient preference.

What is one negative effect of tricyclic antidepressants in patients with coexisting depression and epilepsy?	Tricyclics decrease the seizure threshold
Which tricyclic antidepressants are known to have more anticholinergic effects	Third degree tricyclics (e.g., amitriptyline)
What are examples of other third degree tricyclics antidepressants?	Imipramine Doxepin
Which tricyclic agent is the least sedating?	Desipramine
Which tricyclic is prescribed for enuresis (bed-wetting)?	Imipramine
Which tricyclic is prescribed for obsessive-compulsive disorder?	Clomipramine **Note:** This is the most serotonin-specific tricyclic.
Which tricyclic is the least likely to cause orthostatic hypertension and therefore the best choice for treating an elderly depressed patient with a tricyclic?	Nortriptyline (SSRIs are preferable overall, though)
What is the most common indication for MAOIs (monoamine oxidase inhibitors)?	Treatment of atypical depression
What is the mechanism of action of MAOIs?	They work by inhibiting the mitochondrial enzyme monoamine oxidase which metabolizes norepinephrine, serotonin, and dopamine resulting in a build up of these biogenic amines and their subsequent leakage into the synapse.
What are the names of commonly prescribed MAOIs?	Isocarboxazid Phenelzine Tranylcypromine
What are the common side effects of MAOIs	Sedation Anticholinergic effects Orthostatic hypotension Cardiac conduction disturbances
What other medication must be avoided in patients taking MAOIs?	Pseudoephedrine must be avoided because it can cause hypertensive crisis.

What other substance must be avoided by patients taking MAOIs?

Tyramine, which is found in aged cheeses, beer, certain meats and fish, fava beans, red wine (particularly Chianti), avocados, chocolate, and dairy products. Signs of tyramine ingestions include headache, arrhythmias, and hypertensive crisis.

What is the most popular of the biochemical theories that explain the development of psychosis?

The dopamine hypothesis which cites an increase in dopamine transmission as the cause of delusions, which is supported by evidence that D2 receptors are increased in schizophrenic patients.

What are some pharmacologic agents that cause psychosis?

Amphetamines

Cocaine

L-Dopa

What is the mechanism of action for most typical antipsychotics?

They are dopamine receptor antagonists.

What is the most common problematic side effect of typical antipsychotics?

Extrapyramidal effects/Parkinson's like side effects:

Bradykinesia

Rigidity

Tremor

Acute dystonia

Akathisia

Note: Chronic tardive dyskinesias may also occur.

Which of the extrapyramidal side effects is a flag for caution for future use of typical antipsychotics?

Acute dystonic reaction

Which typical antipsychotics have the most extrapyramidal effects?

Fluphenazine = haloperidol > chlorpromazine > thioridazine

This is correlated with potency/D2 blockade.

Which is the most potent of the typical antipsychotics?

Fluphenazine

What is the mechanism of action of the atypical antipsychotic clozapine?

It acts on dopamine, serotonin, and acetylcholine receptors.

What is the greatest benefit of atypical antipsychotics?	They usually have fewer extrapyramidal side effects than typical antipsychotics.
What is the major side effect to beware of with clozapine?	Agranulocytosis → necessitates weekly or biweekly white blood cells (WBC) monitoring in patients on clozapine therapy.
What is the mechanism of action of the atypical antipsychotic risperidone?	It works by blocking both dopamine and serotonin receptors.
What are other common side effects of antipsychotic therapy?	Amenorrhea Anticholinergic effects Antihistaminergic effects/sedation Photosensitivity Temperature dysregulation Neuroleptic malignant syndrome Blood dyscrasias
What is the cause of amenorrhea in women taking antipsychotics?	Dopamine receptor antagonism
Which pharmacologic agents are used to treat mania associated with bipolar disorder?	Lithium carbonate Lithium citrate Atypical antipsychotics Divalproex sodium Carbamazepine
What are some of the side effects of lithium?	Polyuria → acts as an antidiuretic hormone (ADH) antagonist to cause nephrogenic diabetes insipidus Tremor Hypothyroidism Weight gain Gastrointestinal effects (nausea, vomiting, diarrhea) **Note:** Use of lithium requires close monitoring of serum levels.
Why is lithium contraindicated in pregnant women?	It causes first trimester congenital abnormalities, especially of the heart and associated structures.
How long does it take for lithium to have a therapeutic effect?	2 to 3 weeks

Which anticonvulsants are used to treat bipolar disorder?	Carbamazepine Valproic acid
What type of therapy is used for major depressive order that is refractory to treatment?	Electroconvulsive therapy (ECT)
In what other psychiatric conditions can ECT be used as treatment therapy?	Acute mania Schizophrenia with catatonic symptoms
When does the maximum response to ECT usually occur?	After a 2 to 3-week period over which 5 to 10 treatments are administered.
What are some of the adverse effects of ECT?	Bone fractures → muscle relaxants and general anesthesia will minimize these effects Amnesia
In which patients is ECT contraindicated?	Patients with increased intracranial pressure
How can the amnesia associated with ECT be minimized?	Unilateral electrode placement

CHAPTER 10

Psychotic Disorders

PSYCHOTIC DISORDERS

What is psychosis?

Significant impairment in reality testing (ability to distinguish real from imaginary)

What are the clinical hallmarks of psychosis?

Delusions—fixed false beliefs, despite evidence to the contrary

Hallucinations—usually auditory

Disorganized speech (thought disorder)

Grossly disorganized or catatonic (stupor and bizarre posturing) behavior

What is the difference between a hallucination and an illusion?

An illusion is the misperception of an actual sensory stimulus (e.g., seeing a pool of water on the road ahead during a hot summer day), whereas hallucinations are perceptions in the absence of an external stimulus.

Other than primary psychotic disorders, like schizophrenia, what other types of psychiatric illness often manifest psychotic symptoms?

1. Mood disorders—severe major depression or manic episodes. People who develop psychotic symptoms, do so only during a mood episode and not when their moods are normal (euthymic).
2. Substance use—acute intoxication (especially with cocaine, lysergic acid diethylamide (LSD), phencyclidine (PCP), and amphetamines) or withdrawal (especially alcohol). Anytime a patient has tactile hallucinations, you should think about drugs.

3. Personality disorders—borderline personality disorder may be associated with brief (minutes) periods of psychosis.

   Tip: Watch out for schizoid and schizotypal personality disorders—these people do not become psychotic, but these are usually thrown in as tricks.
4. Cognitive disorders—both delirium and dementia can have psychosis. Often delirium will have visual hallucinations in addition to clouded sensorium.
5. Narcolepsy—may have hypnagogic and hypnopompic hallucinations.

Name the six major primary psychotic disorders.

1. Brief psychotic disorder (<1 month of symptoms)
2. Schizophreniform disorder (1 to 6 months of symptoms)
3. Schizophrenia (>6 months of symptoms)
4. Schizoaffective disorder
5. Delusional disorder
6. Shared psychotic disorder

   Tip: You do not need to know everything about each of the above disorders. Key features, which may be of importance, will be covered later in this chapter.

Schizophrenia

Which of the primary psychotic disorders is the most common?

Schizophrenia. The incidence in the adult population is around 1%.

In addition to the hallmarks of psychosis identified earlier, what other symptoms are commonly present?

Negative symptoms (think *deficits*). These include affective flattening, alienation (social withdrawal), alogia (poverty of speech), and avolition (lack of motivation). In addition to the four hallmarks discussed above, these are the five major diagnostic criteria of schizophrenia.

What are considered the *positive symptoms* of schizophrenia?

Usually this refers to the hallucinations, delusions, bizarre behavior, and thought disorder.

How does the criterion of *disorganized speech,* (also referred to as *thought disorder*) manifest in schizophrenia?

Abnormalities in thought processes and thought formation

Give at least two examples of abnormal thought formation.

1. Word salad—words and phrases are combined together in incoherent manner
2. Neologisms—creation of new words
3. Echolalia—repeating the same word over and over (almost like a mental stutter)
4. Loose associations and flight of ideas—illogical shifting between unrelated or obliquely related topics (also seen in mania)
5. Thought blocking
6. Circumstantial and tangential thought—circumstantial thought eventually gets to the point; tangential never does.

A → B
Normal

A → X → Y → B
Circumstantial

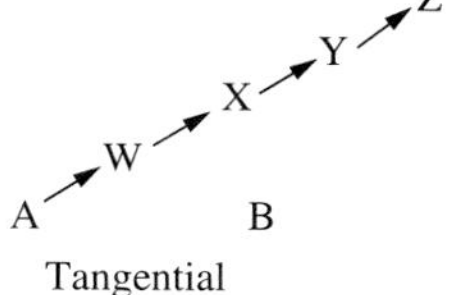

Tangential

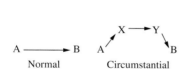

What is meant by the prodromal and residual phases of schizophrenia?

These are periods of time before and after active psychotic periods. These periods are generally characterized by attenuated symptoms of the active phase, e.g., social withdrawal, peculiar behavior, or odd affect.

Tip: During these periods a person would seem strange but would not necessarily meet criteria for *psychotic.*

How long must you have symptoms for before schizophrenia can be diagnosed?

At least 6 months. This includes prodromal and residual phases, but they must have at least 1 month of active symptoms including at least two of the five major types of symptoms. These symptoms must cause some sort of dysfunction.

Does gender affect the development of schizophrenia?

There is no difference in the prevalence of schizophrenia between men and women; however, the age of onset is affected. Men tend to develop it between 15 and 25 years of age and women between 25 and 35 years of age.

What other epidemiological factors are correlated with increased risk of schizophrenia?

Having a first degree relative with schizophrenia increases a patients' risk of schizophrenia tenfold. Being born in the cold winter months or in an area of high population density have also been associated with increased risk (though less so).

What is *downward drift*?

This is the tendency of schizophrenics to be of lower socioeconomic status. It is generally thought that this is due to inability to function well in society, causing a "drift" into lower socioeconomic classes.

What is the *dopamine hypothesis*?

This is the classic understanding of schizophrenia, which attributes the symptoms of schizophrenia to hyperactivity of the dopaminergic system. (Recent research reveals schizophrenia to be much more complex but this will not be considered here.)

Is there any structural brain changes associated with schizophrenia?

Increase in size in the lateral and third ventricles, generalized atrophy of the cortex, and frontal lobe abnormalities are classically associated with schizophrenia.

What are the five major subtypes of schizophrenia?

Paranoid

Residual

Catatonic

Disorganized

Undifferentiated

Which form tends to have the best social functioning?

Paranoid. They also tend to be slightly older at onset, and have prominent hallucinations and delusions, with a lesser component of disorganization.

Which form is the least common?

Catatonic (waxy flexibility may be present). Prior to the development of antipsychotics, this form was more common.

What is the most predictive of overall prognosis?

Level of premorbid function

Overall, schizophrenia is associated with repeated psychotic episodes, and a chronic downhill course. What features are associated with a somewhat better prognosis?

Abrupt onset, female gender, presence of mood symptoms, and old age at onset

Are patients with schizophrenia at risk of suicide?

Yes! Over half of schizophrenics will attempt suicide at some point in their lives, and 10% will die from it.

What is the primary treatment for schizophrenia?

Antipsychotics, which block dopamine in the mesolimbic system.

What is the difference between *typical* and *atypical* antipsychotics?

Typical antipsychotics are older and are primarily useful at treating the positive symptoms of schizophrenia. Side effects include weight gain, sedation, and higher rates of extrapyramidal symptoms (EPS) and tardive dyskinesia (TD).

Atypical antipsychotics are newer, have less EPS and TD, and do a better job treating the negative symptoms (but are still good at treating positive symptoms).

What is EPS?

This includes tremor, rigidity, akathisia (inner restlessness), and acute dystonias (muscle spasm).

How do you treat EPS?

Anticholinergics (e.g., diphenhydramine and benztropine)

How do you treat tardive dyskinesia?

By not causing it in the first place! It is a permanent movement disorder, usually with writhing jerky movement most commonly affecting the mouth area. This is most often seen in older women with long history of antipsychotic use.

What is a potentially fatal side effect of antipsychotic treatment?

Neuroleptic malignant syndrome (NMS). This is an idiosyncratic reaction that is more common in young men. Mortality is nearly 20%.

How does NMS present?

Fever, muscle rigidity, altered mental status, and autonomic instability

What is the first thing you should do if a patient presents to the ER with NMS?

Stop the antipsychotic! Then care is primarily supportive.

Other Psychotic Disorders

What is schizoaffective disorder?

This is similar to schizophrenia but with the addition of mood episodes (like major depressive disorder [MDD] or bipolar disorder). Although counterintuitive, it has a better prognosis than schizophrenia. Schizoaffective disorder may be a totally different illness (or group of illnesses) from schizophrenia.

What are the two types of schizoaffective disorder?

Bipolar

Depressed

How could you differentiate between a primary mood disorder with psychotic features (e.g., MDD with psychosis) from schizoaffective disorder?

A person with an affective disorder that develops psychotic symptoms will not have psychosis in between mood episodes.

Tip: Look at the names! For example, in schizoaffective disorder, the emphasis is on the *schizo*. The primary problem is a psychotic disorder that sometimes has a mood component, whereas in MDD with psychosis, the emphasis is on MDD. The main problem is a mood disorder that when severe, may have a component of psychosis.

What is a delusional disorder?

Patients with delusional disorder tend to have an isolated, fixed, *nonbizarre* delusion (e.g., the Internal Revenue Service [IRS] is after them, or their partner is cheating). People tend to be older (forties) at onset and have relatively preserved functioning outside of the delusion. They are *not* disorganized in thoughts or affect.

CHAPTER 11

Mood Disorders

When do you diagnose major depressive disorder (MDD)?

Episode(s) of depression of at least 2 weeks of duration

How can you recognize a depressive episode?

It is a period of at least 2 weeks, when the patient complains of depressed mood or anhedonia with associated:

↓ concentration

↓ energy

↓ or ↑ sleep

↓ or ↑ appetite

Psychomotor retardation

Agitation

Feelings of worthlessness

Guilt

Recurrent thoughts of death or suicidal ideation

What is anhedonia?

Loss of pleasure in all or almost all activities

What is SIG E CAPS?

It is a mnemonic for depression:

Sleep disturbances (mainly insomnia)

Loss of **I**nterest

Excessive **G**uilt

Loss of **E**nergy

Loss of **C**oncentration

Loss of **A**ppetite

Psychomotor retardation or agitation

Suicidal ideation (or recurrent thoughts of death).

What is the prevalence of MDD?

5% to 12% for men and 10% to 20% for women, with a 2:1 female to male ratio.

What is *masked* depression?	It is when patients deny or seem unaware of the symptoms of depression. This condition can occur in up to 50% of patients.
Does MDD appear at a certain age?	The mean age of onset is 40.
What are the medical conditions that can cause or mimic a depressive episode?	Pancreatic cancer Lung cancer Thyroid dysfunction (particularly hypothyroidism) Pneumonia Mononucleosis Acquired immunodeficiency syndrome (AIDS) Syphilis Parkinson's disease Stroke Multiple sclerosis Lupus Nutritional deficiency Menopause
Are there any medications that can cause depression?	Yes. Reserpine Propranolol Steroids (e.g., prednisone) Methyldopa Interferons (used to treat viral hepatitis)
What is *double* depression?	This term is used when patients meet criteria for MDD and dysthymic disorder
What is dysthymic disorder?	It is an illness where patients feel mildly to moderately depressed for a minimum of 2 years and over the 2-year period the patient has never been without symptoms for more than 2 months. It is not severe enough to meet the criteria for MDD.
How can you differentiate dysthymic disorder from MDD?	Dysthymic disorder lasts for at least 2 years, is longer but with milder symptoms than MDD.

How do you treat depression pharmacologically?

The first-line treatment option is the selective serotonin reuptake inhibitors or SSRIs (see Table 11.1).

Are there any other antidepressants also considered as first-line treatment options?

Yes, there are other antidepressants with different mechanism of action (see Table 11.2).

What are the tricyclics?

Older antidepressants (also known as heterocyclics) are currently considered a second-line treatment option.

Why are the tricyclics a second-line treatment option?

Because they are less tolerable due to their side effect profile and also because they can kill patients if they overdose on them

What are the side effects of the tricyclics?

They include anticholinergic effects (dry mouth, blurred vision, constipation, and confusion), alpha-blocking effects (sedation also caused by antihistaminic effects, orthostatic hypotension, and cardiac arrhythmias), may lower the seizure threshold, are contraindicated in glaucoma, and have to be used with caution in urinary retention (quite a list!!).

What are the most commonly used tricyclics?

Amitriptyline, desipramine, imipramine, and nortriptyline

Are there any other medications to treat depression?

Yes, the monoamine oxidase inhibitors (MAOIs), considered third-line option. MAOIs are *rarely* used any more. The main reason for not using them is due to the diet restrictions and drug-drug interactions.

Why are MAOIs a third-line option?

Because they can cause serotonin syndrome and hypertensive crisis

What is serotonin syndrome?

A clinical entity that consists of hyperthermia, muscle rigidity, and altered mental status. This syndrome is seen when MAOIs are combined with SSRIs (mostly), Demerol, pseudoephedrine, and other medications that can increase serotonin and norepinephrine.

Table 11.1 SSRIs Approved by Food and Drug Administration (FDA) for Treatment of Depression

Generic Name	Brand Name	Side Effects	FDA Indications	Other
Citalopram	Celexa	Nausea, vomiting, headache, sexual side effects, and it can increase anxiety at the beginning of the treatment	Depression	Mildly protein bound, few med-med interactions
Escitalopram	Lexapro	Same	Depression, GAD	Is the isomer of citalopram, very few med-med interactions
Fluoxetine	Prozac	Same	Depression, bulimia, OCD, panic disorder	Highly protein bound, can increase levels of Coumadin and digoxin, long half-life
Paroxetine	Paxil	Same, plus has anticholinergic effects that can cause weight gain, constipation, sedation	Depression, social anxiety disorder, GAD, panic disorder, PTSD, PMDD, OCD	Also highly protein bound, can increase levels of Coumadin and digoxin, short half-life, can cause withdrawal symptoms
Sertraline	Zoloft	Same, can cause more GI side effects	Depression, OCD, PMDD, panic disorder, social anxiety disorder, PTSD	Very few med-med interactions

Abbreviations: GAD, general anxiety disorder; OCD, obsessive-compulsive disorder; PTSD, posttraumatic stress disorder; PMDD, premenstrual dysphoric disorder; PMDD, premenstrual dysphoric disorder; GI, gatrointestinal.

Table 11.2 Other Antidepressants Indicated for the Treatment of Depression

Generic Name	Brand Name	Mechanism of Action	Side Effects	Other
Bupropion	Wellbutrin	Weak inhibitor of the reuptake of serotonin, norepinephrine, and dopamine	Agitation, dry mouth, insomnia, headache, nausea, vomiting, constipation, and tremor	Contraindicated in patients with seizures, bulimia, and anorexia Used to treat sexual side effects caused by SSRIs
Mirtazapine	Remeron	Presynaptic $alpha_2$-adrenergic antagonist (↑norepinephrine and serotonin) also potent antagonist of $5HT_2$ and $5HT_3$	Highly sedating, ↑appetite, ↑weight	Agranulocytosis in 0.1% Also used to ↓ nausea
Trazodone	Desyrel	Weakly inhibits serotonin reuptake Postsynaptically antagonizes $5HT_2$	Highly sedating, orthostatic hypotension Uncommon but can cause priapism (painful erection) and arrhythmias	Used as a sleeping aid
Nefazodone	Serzone	Similar to trazodone	Headache, dry mouth, blurred vision, somnolence, orthostatic hypotension	Causes hepatotoxicity Black-boxed warning from FDA due to risk of liver failure
Venlafaxine	Effexor	Potent inhibitor of serotonin and norepinephrine reuptake, also weak inhibitor of dopamine reuptake	Nausea, dizziness, sexual dysfunction, headache, dry mouth	Can increase blood pressure
Duloxetine	Cymbalta	Similar to venlafaxine	Nausea, dry mouth, constipation, diarrhea, dizziness, insomnia	Also indicated for neuropathic pain

When does a hypertensive crisis occur in the context of MAOI use?	Hypertensive crisis originates when patients who are on MAOIs ingest food rich in tyramine, like wine and cheese.
Are there any other ways to treat depression?	Yes, by using psychotherapy.
What type of psychotherapy is used to treat depression?	Psychodynamic psychotherapy, which focuses on self-understanding and inner conflicts, cognitive-behavioral therapy, which attempts to recognize negative thoughts or behaviors and then tries to change them, and interpersonal therapy, which examines the patient's relationships and their relation to his or her symptoms.
What is electroconvulsive therapy or ECT?	It is the induction of a generalized seizure by applying electric currents to the brain.
When is ECT used?	It is mainly indicated for patients with refractory depression but it can also be used for the treatment of mania.
What are the main side effects of ECT?	Short-term memory loss
When do you diagnose a patient with bipolar disorder (manic-depression)?	When a patient presents with expansive, euphoric, or irritable mood associated with ↑energy, ↓concentration, ↓need to sleep, talkative (clinically called pressured speech), increased activity/goal-directed behavior, racing thoughts, hypersexual, spending large amounts of money, and engaging in risky activities. Most of these symptoms last for at least 1 week.
What is the difference between hypomania and mania?	They present exactly the same but hypomania does not cause significant social and occupational impairment, while mania does. Also, hypomania does *not* result in psychotic symptoms or hospitalization.
What is bipolar I?	It is a diagnosis that is given when a patient presents with a manic episode with or without depressive episodes.

Table 11.3 Mood Stabilizers Approved by the FDA for Treatment of Bipolar Disorder (either I or II)

Generic Name	Brand Name	Side Effects	Levels	Other
Carbamazepine	Tegretol, Carbatrol, Equetro	Drowsiness, dizziness, ataxia, diplopia, blurred vision, sedation, nausea, reversible mild leukopenia, reversible mild increase in *LFTs, tremor, hyponatremia	Are taken when medication reaches steady state, which is in five half-life Half-life is 18 to 55 hours Levels should be drawn in 5 days Normal range: 8 to 12 μg/mL	Induces metabolism of other medications," the great inducer" (↓ their level) Has been associated with hepatitis, severe blood dyscrasias, and rashes
Lamotrigine	Lamictal	Rash may occur in 10% of individuals. Stevens-Johnson syndrome has been reported Headache, diplopia, ataxia, blurred vision, nausea, and vomiting	Rarely used	Is used in the depressed phase of bipolar disorder but approved by FDA for maintenance treatment for bipolar patients to delay time for any mood episode (depressed or manic) Must start low and taper slowly to minimize risk of serious rash!
Lithium	Eskalith	Thirst, increase urination, tremor, weight gain, nausea, vomiting, diarrhea, sedation, edema, goiter or hypothyroidism, ECG changes, sinoatrial node dysfunction, acne, psoriasis, hair loss, benign increase of† WBC and rarely, acute increase in serum creatinine	Half-life: 24 hours Levels should be taken in 5 days Normal range: 0.6 to 1.2 mM	Narrow therapeutic index, can cause toxicity with ↑ sweating, NSAIDs or thiazides diuretics Eating salty chips ↓ lithium levels

(Continued)

Table 11.3 Mood Stabilizers Approved by the FDA for Treatment of Bipolar Disorder (either I or II) (*Continued*)

Generic Name	Brand Name	Side Effects	Levels	Other
Valproic acid	Depakote	Benign elevation of transaminases, nausea, vomiting, diarrhea, sedation, tremor, ataxia, alopecia (hair loss), weight gain, anorexia, thrombocytopenia (↓ platelets)	Half-life is 8 to 12 hours Levels should be taken in 2 to 3 days Normal range: 50 to 150 μg/mL	Inhibits metabolism of other medications (↑ their level) Better than lithium for rapid cycling patients (more than four episodes of mania in 1 year) or mixed episodes (both manic and depressive symptoms)

Abbreviations: ECG, electrocardiogram; NSAIDs, nonsteroidal anti-inflammatory drugs

*Liver function tests

†White blood cells

What is bipolar II?

It is also a diagnosis, given when a patient presents with a major depressive episode and hypomanic episodes, but *no* manic episodes.

Are there any drugs that induce mania?

Yes, steroids and appetite suppressants are the main culprits. Cocaine (crack) and amphetamines may also induce it.

What is cyclothymic disorder?

Many episodes of depression and hypomania occurring for at least 2 years, where depressive episodes are not severe enough to meet criteria for a major depressive episode.

What is the prevalence of bipolar disorder?

Bipolar I has a lifetime prevalence of 0.5% to 1% and a male to female ratio of 1:1. While, bipolar II has a life time prevalence of 0.5% and is more common in women than in men.

CHAPTER 12

Cognitive Disorders

Name the three major categories of cognitive disorders.

Delirium

Dementia

Amnestic disorders

DELIRIUM

What is delirium?

Delirium is a *disturbance of consciousness* and attention that usually develops over a short period of time. The confusion and memory impairment is not better accounted for by a preexisting dementia.

What causes delirium?

Most often it is the result of a general medical condition, but it may also be due to substance intoxication or withdrawal. Almost any medical condition can cause delirium, especially in the elderly, i.e., metabolic derangements, infections, head trauma, and so forth. Often delirium is multifactorial.

While most substances of abuse can cause delirium with acute intoxication, which three are most likely to cause delirium related to withdrawal?

Alcohol (delirium tremens), benzodiazepines, and barbiturates.

What factors predispose to delirium?

Acute medical illness

Age—elderly and young children

Preexisting brain damage—dementia, cerebrovascular disease, tumor

A history of delirium

How common is delirium?

Very common! Roughly 15% to 20% of general hospital patients will have an episode of delirium. In patients over the age of 65, the prevalence can be as high as 30%!

Clinically, what is the hallmark of delirium?

Altered level of consciousness (especially attention and level of arousal). It typically develops over a period of hours to days and mental status alterations *wax and wane* during the day, with periods of lucidity.

In addition to alterations in consciousness, what other features are often found in a patient with delirium?

Altered sleep-wake cycle

Perceptual disturbance

Impaired memory and orientation

Nocturnal worsening of symptoms

Psychomotor agitation

How do you test for delirium?

You cannot. There is no test that is definitive for delirium. Electroencephalogram (EEG) may show nonspecific changes such as diffuse slowing.

How do you treat delirium?

Treat the cause. The medical "workup" in delirium is really just a hunt for the cause.

Tip: Think of delirium like a fever. The fever is not the primary problem; what ever is causing the fever is the problem!

While identifying and treating the cause of a delirium, how do you manage a delirious patient?

Orient the patient frequently and place him in a brightly lit room during the day. Low doses of antipsychotics, like haloperidol or risperidone can be helpful for agitation and hallucinations. Small doses of benzodiazepines can also help with agitation (use benzodiazepines sparingly as they can worsen confusion and/or disinhibit the patient!).

DEMENTIA

What is the core symptom of dementia?

Memory impairment

In order to diagnose dementia, what must be present in addition to memory impairment?

At least one of the following:
- Aphasia (language and naming problems)
- Apraxia (impaired ability to do learned motor tasks, like using objects)
- Agnosia (difficulty recognizing or identifying objects)
- Disturbance of executive function (the ability to plan, organize and carry out tasks, judgment)

How does dementia differ from the normal memory changes of aging?

As we age, we are less able to learn new information, and we process information at a slower speed. However, these changes do not normally interfere with the basic functioning.

When diagnosing dementia, what other disorders in your differential are key to rule out?

It is crucial that you not miss a delirium or a depression. In the elderly, it is not uncommon for them to report multiple memory complaints. If you misdiagnose this as dementia, you will miss a potentially reversible cause of memory impairment. Likewise, if you miss a delirium, you may miss a potentially serious medical problem. Additionally, there are several potentially reversible causes of dementia that you should look for, including neurosyphilis, B12, thiamine and folate deficiencies, and normal pressure hydrocephalus.

What is the prevalence of dementia?

Incidence/prevalence increases with age. The prevalence is approximately 1.5 % in those over 65 years of age. The prevalence increases to 20% after age 85.

What is the most common type of dementia?

Alzheimer's represents about 50% to 60% of dementias. The second most common form is vascular dementia (formerly multi-infarct dementia)

Others include front temporal (Pick's and Creutzfeldt-Jakob), Parkinson's, Huntington's, and human immunodeficiency virus (HIV) dementias.

What is the classical clinical course for Alzheimer's disease?

Slow, gradual onset of memory loss and cognitive impairment (often there are problems with judgment, mood symptoms, and behavioral disturbances as well). The disease is progressive and death usually occurs within 3 years after diagnosis (new data!).

How does this differ from the course of vascular dementia?

Vascular dementia classically has a stepwise decline, as opposed to the slow and steady decline in Alzheimer's. Onset of deficits may be abrupt, and with good control of cardiovascular risk factors the course may remain relatively stable.

What are the major risk factors for Alzheimer's?

Age, family history, Apo E4 allele, and Down syndrome

On postmortem exam, what changes are normally seen in the brain of an Alzheimer's patient?

Neurofibrillary tangles and senile (amyloid) plaques.

What areas of the brain show cell loss in Alzheimer's?

While there is also often global cortical atrophy, neuronal degeneration is classically in the cholinergic neurons of the nucleus basalis of Meynert.

What class of medications is used to slow the progression of Alzheimer's?

Acetylcholinesterase inhibitors. Since the cholinergic cells are being lost, these medications help increase the presence of acetylcholine in the brain by inhibiting the breakdown of this neurotransmitter.

Table 12.1 Delirium vs. Dementia

	Delirium	Dementia
Onset	Develops quickly (hours to days)	Develops over weeks to years
Key feature	Impaired attention and level of consciousness	Impaired memory with normal level of consciousness
Course	Fluctuates within the course of a day with lucid periods. Worsens at night	Usually stable within a day. May worsen at night (sundowning)
Occurrence	Most common in elderly and young children	Increases with age
Psychiatric symptoms	Hallucinations and delusions may be present	Hallucinations and delusions may be present
Physical findings	Abnormal EEG Acute medical illness	Normal EEG No acute medical illness
Prognosis	Symptoms tend to resolve with treatment of underlying cause	Usually progressive

AMNESTIC SYNDROMES

How do amnestic syndromes differ from dementia?

In amnestic syndromes the disturbance of function is isolated to memory, while other cognitive functions remain relatively intact (unlike dementia).

Which brain structures are affected in amnestic syndromes?

The bilateral mediotemporal structures (e.g., mammillary bodies, hippocampus, fornix)

Damage to mediotemporal structures is associated with what vitamin deficiency?

Thiamine deficiency. Often this is related with chronic alcohol abuse (Korsakoff's syndrome)

Name at least two other etiologies of amnestic syndromes

Traumatic brain injury

Herpes encephalitis

Cerebrovascular disease

Hypoxia

CHAPTER 13

Anxiety Disorders

What are the most prevalent psychiatric disorders?	Anxiety disorders
What are the major types of anxiety disorders?	Generalized anxiety disorder (GAD) Panic disorder Social phobia Specific phobia Obsessive-compulsive disorder Agoraphobia Post-traumatic stress disorder (PTSD) Acute stress disorder (ASD)
What is the most prominent feature of all anxiety disorders?	The presence of a sense of impending doom or threat
What differentiates anxiety disorders from healthy anxiety?	Anxiety out of proportion to actual threat which causes significant distress or impairment
How do you define GAD?	Chronic, excessive worry about several general life events
What are the symptoms of GAD?	Restlessness Tension Insomnia Irritability Decreased concentration
How long should symptoms last to be diagnosed as GAD?	6 months
What is the male:female ratio of GAD prevalence?	1:2

What are important nonpsychiatric differentials to consider for GAD?

Substance-induced anxiety
Substance withdrawal anxiety
Pheochromocytoma
Hyperthyroidism
Electrolyte abnormalities

What is the initial pharmacological treatment for GAD?

Selective serotonin reuptake inhibitor (SSRI)
Venlafaxine
Buspirone
Mirtazapine

PANIC DISORDER

What are the symptoms of a panic attack?

Anxiety
Palpitations
Sweating
Dizziness
Trembling
Shortness of breath
Chest pain
Nausea
Feeling of choking
Chills
Fear of dying

What characterizes panic disorder?

Periods of intense fear with *spontaneous* panic attacks
Impending doom
Anxiety about future attacks

What differentiates panic attacks from panic disorders?

Panic attacks are the initial event. A panic disorder develops when the patient has recurrent attacks and has anticipatory fear.

What is the male:female ratio for panic disorder?

1:3

What is the age of onset of panic disorder?

Mid-twenties

Is family history of panic disorders relevant?

Yes, evidence does support an upregulation of adrenergic output responsible for stimulating anxiety centers in the brain which predisposes certain people to panic attacks.

What are the most common psychiatric sequelae of panic attacks?	Agoraphobia. Patients have anticipatory fear which prevents them from venturing outside alone.
What is the most effective psychotherapy for panic disorder?	Cognitive behavioral therapy including relaxation techniques
What is the pharmacologic treatment of panic disorder?	SSRIs (first-line) Tricyclic antidepressant (TCA), monoamine oxidase inhibitors (MAOIs) (second-line)
What are the important nonpsychiatric differential diagnoses for panic disorders?	Arrhythmias Angina Hypoxia Hyperthyroidism Substance induced intoxication or withdrawal

OBSESSIVE-COMPULSIVE DISORDER

What is the main characteristic of obsessive-compulsive disorder (OCD)?	Recurrent obsessive thoughts, impulses, or images that cause anxiety and/or compulsive behaviors.
What are the symptoms of OCD?	Anxiety Nervousness Depression Social isolation Fear of dirt Excessive cleaning or washing Fear of harm to self or loved ones Excessive checking
What differentiates OCD from obsessive-compulsive personality disorder (OCPD)?	Patients with OCD are aware that anxiety is not healthy and acknowledge they have a problem. Patients with OCPD are not aware of their condition. OCD is a Diagnostic and Statistical Manual of Mental Disorders—Fourth Edition (DSM-IV) Axis I disorder whereas OCPD is an Axis II disorder.
What is the male:female ratio for OCD?	1:1
What is the age of onset of OCD?	Late adolescence to early adulthood

What is a common psychiatric diagnosis associated with OCD?	Tourette's syndrome **Note:** It is common for patients with Tourette's to have OCD, but it is *not* nearly as common for patients with OCD to have Tourette's.
What is the most effective psychotherapy for OCD?	Behavioral therapy (exposure-response prevention, flooding, thought stopping)
What is the pharmacologic treatment of OCD?	High dose SSRI (first-line treatment) Clomipramine (second-line treatment)
What are the important differential diagnoses for OCD?	Specific phobia GAD Body dimorphic disorder Trichotillomania
What are the characteristics of obsessions and compulsions present in persons with OCD?	Obsessions and compulsions are time consuming, interrupt daily living and function, and cause obvious distress.

SOCIAL PHOBIA

What are the symptoms of a social phobia?	Fear of social situations Anxiety Palpitations Sweating Headache Restlessness
What characterizes social phobias?	Excessive, irrational fear of public or social situations, in which the patient could be scrutinized for his or her performance
What differentiates social phobias from specific phobias?	Social phobias involve fear of public situations where scrutiny could occur. On the other hand, specific phobias involve fear of specific objects or situations not associated with scrutiny.
What is the male:female ratio for social phobia?	1:1
What is the age of onset of social phobias?	Adolescence following childhood shyness

What are the most common social phobias?
Fear of public speaking
Fear of public performances
Fear of answering questions in class

What is the most effective psychotherapy for social phobias?
Cognitive behavioral therapy including relaxation techniques

What is the pharmacologic treatment of social phobias?
SSRIs (first-line treatment)
MAOIs
Beta-blockers

What are the important differential diagnoses for social phobia?
Specific phobias
Panic disorder
OCD

POST-TRAUMATIC STRESS DISORDER

What is the main characteristic of post-traumatic stress disorder (PTSD)?
Nightmares/flashbacks
Intrusive thoughts
Sleep disturbances
Social dysfunction secondary to physical and/or psychological trauma

What are the symptoms of PTSD?
Nightmares
Insomnia
Flashbacks
Irritability
Hypervigilance
Increased startle response
Survivor guilt
Personality change

What differentiates PTSD from acute stress disorder?
Patients with PTSD have symptoms for greater than 1 month that can begin more than 1 month after the traumatic event occurs. Patients with acute stress disorder have symptoms lasting from 2 days to 1 month which begin within 1 month of traumatic event.

What differentiates PTSD from adjustment disorder?
PTSD involves life-threatening events (rape, war, and so forth)
Adjustment disorders involve nonlife-threatening events (divorce, death of others)

What is the male:female ratio for PTSD?	1:2
What is the age of onset of PTSD?	Young adulthood **Note:** There may be a late onset of PTSD if the stressful situation which triggers this disorder occurs later on in life.
How is PTSD classified?	Acute PTSD: Symptoms last less than 3 months Chronic PTSD: Symptoms last greater than 3 months Delayed-onset PTSD: Symptoms begin more than 6 months after the life-threatening event
What is the most effective psychotherapy for PTSD?	Cognitive-behavioral therapy (CBT) and support groups
What is the pharmacologic treatment of PTSD?	SSRIs (first-line treatment) Mood stabilizers
What are important differential diagnoses for PTSD?	Acute stress disorder Adjustment disorder OCD Malingering

SPECIFIC PHOBIA

What are the symptoms of a specific phobia?	Fear of specific situations Anxiety Palpitations Sweating Headache Restlessness
What characterizes specific phobias?	Excessive, irrational fear of specific objects or situations
What differentiates specific phobias from social phobias?	Specific phobias involve fear of specific objections or situations not associated with being scrutinized.
What is the male:female ratio for specific phobia?	1:2
What is the age of onset of specific phobias?	Mostly childhood but can begin at anytime

What are the most common types of specific phobias?

Animals
Storms
Heights
Illness
Injury

What is the most effective psychotherapy for specific phobias?

Flooding
Gradual desensitization
Hypnosis
CBT

What is the pharmacologic treatment of specific phobias?

Benzodiazepines for certain phobias such as flying

What are important differential diagnoses for specific phobias?

Social phobia
OCD
GAD
Panic disorder

ADJUSTMENT DISORDER WITH ANXIETY

What is the main characteristic of adjustment disorder with anxiety?

Emotional or behavioral symptoms associated with an identifiable stressor

During what time period should the symptoms present after stressor occurs?

Within 3 months of initial stressor

When should symptoms of adjustment disorder with anxiety resolve?

Within 6 months of initial symptoms

What are common causes of adjustment disorder?

Divorce
Relocation
Attending a new school

What should be ruled out before diagnosing adjustment disorders?

Bereavement
Any Axis I diagnosis

How does adjustment disorder with anxiety present?

Occupational impairment
Social impairment
Scholastic impairment

What are important differential diagnoses?

Bereavement
Major depressive disorder
Acute stress disorder
PTSD

CHAPTER 14

Somatoform Disorders

What is the primary difference between somatoform and factitious disorders?

Somatoform disorders are unconscious manifestations of disease, whereas factitious disorders are consciously derived by the patient for primary or secondary gain.

Which gender is more prevalent in the somatoform disorders?

Female

What are the primary types of somatoform disorders?

Somatization disorder

Conversion disorder

Hypochondriasis

Body dysmorphic disorder

Pain disorder

What is the age of onset of somatoform disorders?

Somatic complaints must begin prior to age 30

Note: This requirement is *only* for somatization disorder.

Are there any physical exam findings which are common in somatoform disorders?

No. Disease etiology must be ruled out in these patients; however, there is no medical condition that can account for their symptoms.

How long must these symptoms be present for a diagnosis of a somatoform disorder?

These disorders often span over a few years, and they must cause significant impairment in the patient's personal, social, or occupational activities.

Should patients with somatoform disorders be told that they are imagining their symptoms?

No. Supportive treatment with suggestions that psychotherapy may alleviate their distress is associated with a better prognosis.

What are the primary types of factitious disorders?

Munchausen syndrome

Munchausen by proxy

Which gender is more prevalent in factitious disorders?	Female
What occupation has the highest prevalence of factitious disorders?	Health-care workers
What is primary gain?	Receiving a psychological benefit from assuming the sick role
What is secondary gain?	Receiving an external benefit from assuming the sick role (e.g., avoiding jail, receiving disability)
Are patients with factitious disorders aware of the false nature of their somatic complaints?	Yes. This is the distinguishing characteristic between factitious and somatoform disorders. Often these patients create their symptoms or frankly lie.

MALINGERING

What is the primary characteristic of malingering?	Intentional production of symptoms for secondary gain
How is malingering different from factitious disorder?	The goal of malingering is to obtain a concrete or material gain.
What are common scenarios in which malingering is often seen?	Individuals wanting to avoid jail time or military recruitment, seeking financial compensation, and so forth
Which gender is most prevalent in malingering?	Males
What is Ganser syndrome?	A variant of malingering in which patients give ridiculous answers to questions in order to avoid responsibility for their actions.
In what populations is Ganser syndrome most commonly seen?	Prison inmates

MUNCHAUSEN SYNDROME

What is the primary characteristic of factitious disorder?	Intentional simulation of illness for primary gain
How is factitious disorder different from malingering?	The goal of factitious disorder is to assume the sick role.

What disease presentations are seen in factitious disorder?	Hematuria (from adding blood to urine or from the use of anticoagulants) and hypoglycemia (from insulin injection)
What laboratory finding would indicate self-injection of insulin?	Low C peptide level
What are common behaviors seen in patients with factitious disorder?	Requests for analgesics Extensive knowledge of medical terminology Eager desire to undergo medical procedures and operations Traveling to different locations, hospitals, emergency rooms, and so forth
What are common clinical presentations of patients with factitious disorder?	Patients often have dramatic histories with extensive details about their symptoms.
What is the appropriate treatment for factitious disorder?	Recognition and confrontation in a nonaccusatory manner
What is the prevalence of factitious disorder?	0.5% to 0.8%—very difficult to determine
Which gender is most commonly seen in factitious disorder?	Females
What is the primary characteristic of factitious disorder by proxy?	Intentional simulation of illness in another person
Who is the most common perpetrator seen in factitious disorder by proxy?	A parent (most often a mother) often stimulating illness in her child.
What is the treatment for factitious disorder by proxy?	Same as in factitious disorder, however, if a child is involved, the case should be managed as child abuse and reported to the appropriate agencies.

SOMATIZATION DISORDER

What are the diagnostic criteria of complaints seen in somatization disorder?	Patients must manifest four pain, two gastrointestinal, one sexual, and one neurological symptoms, all of which cannot be fully explained by medical etiology.

What are common patterns of behaviors seen in these patients?

These patients often have had multiple exploratory surgeries and visit multiple doctors.

Can the symptoms occur in the presence of a true medical condition?

Yes, however, the complaints will often be in excess of what would be normally expected.

What is the prevalence of somatization disorders in the United States?

0.2% to 2% in women and less than 0.2% in men

What are risk factors for somatization disorder?

High socioeconomic status

History of abusive and failed relationships

Family history of somatization

What is the most common first manifestation of this disorder in women?

Complaints relating to menses

What is the treatment for somatization disorders?

Regular brief appointments with the primary care provider are often useful in reassuring these patients. Unnecessary lab tests or procedures should not be performed. In addition, psychotherapy may be used.

CONVERSION DISORDER

From which body system are complaints derived from in conversion disorders?

Neurological (motor and/or sensory)

What are the most common manifestations seen?

Sudden onset of blindness

Paralysis

Paresthesias

Seizures

What are common findings on physical exam of these patients?

Abnormalities do not have anatomical distribution and neurological exam is normal

What is a common association with the onset or exacerbation of symptoms?

Often stressful life events precede the development of symptoms

What medical disorder can present similarly to a conversion disorder?

Multiple sclerosis

What percentage of individuals diagnosed with a conversion disorder in fact have a true neurological condition?

Estimated to range from one-third (33%) to half (50%)

Do patients with true conversion disorders sustain injury as a result of their condition?

No. Patients with sudden onset of blindness do not run into objects, and those with paralysis may still inadvertently move when distracted.

Are patients with conversion disorder distressed over their condition?

No. These patients are often calm regarding their pseudoneurological deficits, termed *la belle indifference.* **Note:** This is not diagnostic of conversion disorder.

Do patients with conversion disorder intentionally derive primary or secondary gain from their symptoms?

No

What is the prognosis and duration of symptoms seen in conversion disorders?

Symptoms typically remit within 2 weeks, with favorable prognosis seen in paralysis and blindness, and a poor prognosis associated with seizures

What is the treatment for conversion disorders?

Relaxation techniques are standard; additionally anxiolytics such as benzodiazepines can occasionally be used. Reassurance that the symptoms will improve usually results in resolution of the symptoms (self-limiting), however, conversion disorder often reoccurs later.

HYPOCHONDRIASIS

What is the main characteristic of hypochondriasis?

Preoccupation with having a serious disease, despite medical reassurance of health status

Are there true physical symptoms seen in this disorder?

Yes, however, the symptoms are misinterpreted by the patient as being of a greater significance.

What are the most common presenting symptoms seen in hypochondriasis?

Nausea

Abdominal pain

Chest pain

Palpitations

Is there a gender predominance seen in hypochondriasis?
No, men and women are equally affected.

What are common associations with the development of hypochondriasis?
Often the person has experienced serious illness in childhood or knows someone who has died or suffered through a serious medical condition

What are common behaviors seen in these patients?
Doctor shopping is common, as these patients are resistant to suggestions that there is no significant medical etiology to their symptoms

What is the prevalence of hypochondriasis?
1% to 5%

What is the treatment for hypochondriasis?
Group therapy and frequent reassurance with regular but brief visits to primary care physician

BODY DYSMORPHIC DISORDER

What is the main characteristic of body dysmorphic disorder?
Preoccupation with a defect in physical appearance

Is the defect always imagined by the patient?
No. In some patients the defect may be imagined, but in others an exaggeration of a true physical feature may be present.

What are the two components of body dysmorphic disorder?
Perceptual and attitudinal. Perceptual relates to the accuracy of the individual's body. Attitudinal relates to the feelings the person has toward his or her body

What are risk factors for the development of body dysmorphic disorder?
Family history of a mood disorder or obsessive-compulsive disorder

Where do these patients often present?
Often these patients present to dermatologist and plastic surgeons

What are the most common features viewed as defective in these patients?
Facial features

Hair

Body build

What is the most common comorbid psychiatric disorder associated with body dysmorphic disorder?
Depression

What are some common behaviors seen in this disorder?

Excessive grooming

Avoidance of mirrors

Excessive exercise

Avoidance of public activities

What other diagnoses must be considered in the differential?

Anorexia nervosa

Gender identity disorder

Narcissistic personality disorder

Do surgical procedures and alterations tend to improve the patient's view of his or her *physical defect*?

No. These treatments tend to worsen the disorder, leading to intensified or new preoccupations with physical appearance.

What is the recommended treatment for body dysmorphic disorder?

Antidepressants (such as selective serotonin reuptake inhibitors [SSRIs]) (only if comorbid mental illnesses such as depression or anxiety are present) and cognitive behavioral therapy.

CHAPTER 15

Personality Disorders

What is personality?

Personality is "the set of characteristics that defines the behavior, thoughts, and emotions of individuals."

What constitutes a personality disorder?

Personality disorders occur when a particular feature or trait of an individual's personality becomes either inflexible (as in obsessive-compulsive personality disorder) or maladaptive (as in histrionic personality disorder). The second caveat to this definition is that as a result of this feature or trait there is "impairment in social or occupational functioning or subjective distress."

Which axis of the Diagnostic and Statistical Manual of Mental Disorders—Fourth Edition (DSM-IV) do personality disorder diagnoses fall under?

They are Axis II diagnoses

Which personality disorders fall under cluster A?

Paranoid, schizoid, and schizotypal

What is the common theme among cluster A disorders?

They are considered odd or eccentric traits.

SCHIZOID

How is schizoid personality disorder most often described?

Patients have "a pervasive pattern of detachment from social relationships and a restricted range of expression of emotions in interpersonal settings."

What are the symptoms of schizoid personality disorder?

No desire or enjoyment of close relationships

Choice of solitary activities

Little interest in having sexual experiences

Enjoyment of few activities

Lack of close friends

Apparent indifference

Emotional coldness/detachment/flattened affect

PARANOID

How is paranoid personality disorder defined?

Paranoid personality disorder involves a "pervasive and unwarranted suspicion and mistrust of people, hypersensitivity to others, and an inability to deal with feelings."

What are the symptoms of paranoid personality disorder?

Suspicion of exploitation or deceitfulness on the part of others

Preoccupation with unjustified doubts

Reluctance to confide in others

Reading hidden demeanings or threatening meanings into benign remarks or events

Persistently bearing grudges

Perception of attacks on his or her character or reputation to which he or she reacts quickly/angrily

Recurrent suspicions

What is the best treatment for paranoid personality disorder?

Psychotherapy and possibly antipsychotic medications to manage agitation and paranoia (overt delusions are not usually seen)

SCHIZOTYPAL

How is schizotypal personality disorder defined?

Patients with schizotypal personality disorder are usually described as strange or odd in behavior, appearance, and/or thinking. They often look to be schizophrenic, but have no history of psychosis.

What are the symptoms of schizotypal personality disorder?

Ideas of reference

Odd beliefs/magical thinking/believe that they have "special powers"

Unusual perceptual experiences

Odd thinking and speech

Suspiciousness/paranoia

Inappropriate/constricted affect

Odd behavior/appearance

Lack of close friends

Excessive social anxiety

Which personality disorders fall under cluster B?

Histrionic, narcissistic, antisocial, and borderline

What is the common theme among cluster B disorders?

They are described as dramatic, emotional, and erratic.

What other psychiatric diagnoses do patients with cluster B disorders often carry?

Mood disorders are quite prevalent, as well as somatization disorders, and substance abuse/dependence

How is antisocial personality disorder defined?

Patients with antisocial personality disorder have a long history of continuous, chronic antisocial behavior in which they violate the rights of others. This history can be seen as early as childhood.

What prior childhood diagnosis must have been present in order to be diagnosed with antisocial personality disorder as an adult?

Conduct disorder

How are patients with antisocial personality disorder usually described?

Charming, but manipulative. They often have a history of criminal activities and many have a history of substance abuse. They show absolutely no remorse for their actions when other people are harmed.

What is the best treatment of antisocial personality disorder?	Group therapy with setting of boundaries for behavior, selective serotonin reuptake inhibitors (SSRIs), and treatment of underlying substance abuse/misuse if present. These individuals are very refractory to treatment due to their lying, manipulation, and secondary gain (avoidance of prison, work, money, and so forth).
How is borderline personality disorder defined?	Borderline personality disorder involves the primary feature of instability. This is seen in terms of the patient's self-image, interpersonal relationships, and mood. (Think Glenn Close's character in *Fatal Attraction.*)
What defense mechanism is prevalent in patients with borderline personality disorder?	Splitting—e.g., people are either all good or all bad
What are the symptoms of borderline personality disorder?	Frantic efforts to avoid real or imagined abandonment Unstable or intense interpersonal relationships Identity disturbance, impulsivity Recurrent suicidal behavior Self-mutilating behavior Marked reactivity of mood Chronic feelings of emptiness Inappropriate/intense anger Lack of control of anger Transient stress-related paranoid ideation
What are the most prevalent symptoms of borderline personality disorder?	Unstable relationships and mood/affect lability
What developmental characteristics are often present in patients with borderline personality disorder?	Many were severely abused as children
What is the best treatment for borderline personality disorder?	Psychotherapy plus mood stabilization with either antidepressants, carbamazepine, or valproate. Patients may also require short-term antipsychotics for treatment of psychosis.

What drug class should be avoided in patients with borderline personality disorder?

Benzodiazepines, because of addictive potential and mortality with overdose

How is narcissistic personality disorder described?

Narcissistic personality disorder is defined as a grandiose sense of self-importance along with extreme sensitivity to criticism. These patients have "little ability to sympathize with others, and are more concerned about appearance than substance." (Think Bill Murray's character in *Groundhog Day* or Jack Nicholson in *As Good As It Gets.*)

What are the symptoms of narcissistic personality disorder?

Grandiose sense of self importance/ exaggeration of achievements and talents

Preoccupations with ideals of success, power, brilliance, beauty, and so forth. Belief that he or she is special or unique, and can only be understood or appreciated by high status individuals

Sense of entitlement

Lacks empathy for others

Manipulative

Jealous

Believes others envy him or her

Arrogant

What other psychiatric conditions are associated with narcissistic personality disorder?

Mood disorders and other cluster B traits

What is the best treatment of narcissistic personality disorder?

Psychotherapy (either group or individual)

How is histrionic personality disorder described?

Histrionic personality disorder can be identified by the flamboyant/ attention-seeking behaviors of patients. They are extremely emotional, and may present as very attractive and seductive. (Think Scarlett O'Hara in *Gone with the Wind.*)

What are the symptoms of histrionic personality disorder?

Persistent need to be the center of attention

Inappropriately sexual/seductive/provocative

Insincere

Impressionistic

Melodramatic

Exaggeration of importance

Suggestibility/easy to manipulate

What other psychiatric disorders are often associated with histrionic personality disorder?

Mood disorders and somatization disorders

What is the best treatment of histrionic personality disorder?

Psychotherapy and antidepressants for underlying mood disorders

Which personality disorders fall under cluster C?

Avoidant, dependent, and obsessive-compulsive

What is the common theme among cluster C disorders?

They tend to be anxious and fearful

How is avoidant personality disorder often described?

Individuals with avoidant personality disorder are often shy and timid. They are very self-critical and have low self-esteem.

What other personality disorder may avoidant personality disorder be mistaken for?

Schizoid personality disorder

How can avoidant personality disorder and schizoid personality disorder be differentiated?

Patients with avoidant personality disorder want to have interpersonal relationships but are afraid of rejection; whereas, schizoid personality disorder patients do not wish to have relationships with others.

What are the symptoms of avoidant personality disorder?

Avoidance of activities that involve interaction with others

Fear of intimacy/lack of intimate relationships

Preoccupation with criticism or rejection

Low self-esteem

Reluctance to become involved in new activities

What other psychiatric conditions are often seen in patients with avoidant personality disorder?

Social phobia, specific phobia, and agoraphobia

What is the best treatment of avoidant personality disorder?

Psychotherapy and assertiveness training

How is dependent personality disorder described?

Patients are passive and may let others direct their lives and make important decisions. (Think Bill Murray's character in *What about Bob?*)

What are the symptoms of dependent personality disorder?

Inability to make decisions

Refusal to assume responsibility

Difficulty initiating projects

Need for excessive nurturing and support

Feelings of discomfort and helplessness when alone/persistent need to be in a relationship

Unrealistic fears

What other psychiatric disorders are common in individuals with dependent personality disorder?

Depression and anxiety disorders

What is the best treatment for dependent personality disorder?

Psychotherapy and assertiveness training

How is obsessive-compulsive personality disorder described?

Individuals have extreme perfectionist tendencies and inflexibility. They may have difficulty relating to or empathizing with others. (Think about your classmates.)

How does obsessive-compulsive personality disorder differ from obsessive-compulsive disorder?

Individuals with obsessive-compulsive personality disorder do not have intrusive thoughts (obsessions) or actions that they must carry out to relieve the anxiety provoked by those thoughts (compulsions). They are, on the other hand, very regimented in the way they like to do things and pay very close attention to details.

What are the symptoms of obsessive-compulsive personality disorder?

Preoccupation with rules/details/organizations—often to the point that they have difficulty seeing/understanding the "big picture"

Perfectionistic

Excessive devotion to work and productivity

Inflexible

Pack rats

Reluctant to delegate to others

Cheap/frugal

Rigid

Stubborn

What is the best treatment for obsessive-compulsive personality disorder?

Psychotherapy

CHAPTER 16

Dissociative Disorders

What are the primary characteristics of dissociative disorders?	1. Sudden memory loss of time periods, events, and people 2. Detachment from one's self 3. Derealization 4. Blurred sense of identity
What are the four major dissociative disorders?	Dissociative amnesia Dissociative fugue Dissociative identity disorder Depersonalization disorder
Which conditions are included in the differential diagnosis of dissociative disorders?	Substance abuse Seizure disorders Head injury Post-traumatic stress disorder Malingering
Which disorder is associated with an inability to remember important personal information?	Dissociative amnesia
Which group of people is most likely to suffer from dissociative amnesia?	Young adult females
What is the primary trigger for dissociative amnesia?	Often follows a psychologically traumatic event
What treatment modality is used for dissociative amnesia?	Psychotherapy
What disorder is associated with an inability to remember important personal information and wandering away from home to adopt a new identity?	Dissociative fugue
How long does it normally take for the amnesia to resolve in a person who is experiencing dissociative amnesia or dissociative fugue?	Minutes or days; may last for years

What treatment modality is used for dissociative fugue?	Supportive psychotherapy Hypnosis Drug-assisted interviews
What pharmacological agent is used in drug-assisted interviews?	Sodium amobarbital
Which disorder is associated with a person having multiple personalities?	Dissociative identity disorder
How many personalities are commonly found in a person with dissociative identity disorder?	5 to 10 personalities
Which gender is most likely to develop dissociative identity disorder?	Females
What conditions may dissociative identity disorder resemble?	Borderline personality disorder Schizophrenia
What treatment modality is used for dissociative identity disorder?	Psychotherapy and hypnotherapy
Which disorder is associated with repeated episodes of detachment and unreality about one's own body, social situation, or the environment (derealization)?	Depersonalization disorder
What treatment modality is used for depersonalization disorder?	Psychotherapy; pharmacologic interventions utilized for associated anxiety or depression

CHAPTER 17

Obesity and Eating Disorders

How is obesity diagnosed?

Obesity is diagnosed when a person's body weight is greater than 20% above his or her ideal body weight for a given height. This can also be defined as a body mass index (BMI) greater than 30.

How is BMI calculated?

The BMI is the weight in kilograms (kg) divided by the square of the height in meters (weight/height^2).

What health problems are increased in obese people?

Cardiovascular disease

Cancer

Osteoarthritis

Diabetes mellitus

Chronic obstructive pulmonary disease (COPD)/respiratory disease

What is the prevalence of obesity among adults in the United States?

An estimated 30% of U.S. adults aged 20 years and older—over 60 million people—are obese, defined as having a BMI of 30 or higher.

What are nonmedical risk factors for obesity?

Genetics

Low socioeconomic status

Sedentary lifestyle

What is the number one predictor of adult obesity?

Childhood obesity

What is the best treatment for obesity?

A combination of diet and exercise

What are the diagnostic criteria for anorexia nervosa?

Severe weight loss (greater than 15% of body weight)

Refusal to eat

Amenorrhea (must be present)

Intense fear of gaining weight

Disturbance in the way weight is perceived

What are the associated physical or biological findings in anorexia nervosa?

Lanugo

Melanosis coli

Anemia

Leukopenia

Electrolyte imbalance

How is amenorrhea defined?

Absence of a menstrual period for at least three cycles

What is lanugo?

Fine, downy body hair, especially seen on the trunk

What is melanosis coli?

Blackened areas on the colon, seen with laxative abuse

What is a long-term risk of anorexia?

Early onset and generalized increased risk of osteoporosis

What are some of the warning signs of anorexia?

Excessive dieting, exercise, use of laxatives/diuretics/enemas

Abnormal eating habits

Body image disorder/body dysmorphic disorder

Fear of becoming fat

Decreased libido

What is the typical profile of a patient with anorexia?

Anorexia is most commonly seen in adolescent to young adult females who are very high achieving (either academically, athletically, or both). There is often a lot of conflict within the family, sometimes described as a controlling or overly protective mother.

Do patients with anorexia typically have coexisting mood disorders?

No, they usually have normal mood (they can definitely have associated depression, however).

What is the best treatment for anorexia nervosa?

The patient should be hospitalized to restore nutrition and electrolytes. Psychotherapy should also be considered.

What are the diagnostic criteria for bulimia nervosa?	Repeated vomiting or laxative abuse Repetitive binge eating Self-evaluation influenced by body shape and weight
What are common associated findings in persons with bulimia nervosa?	Erosion of tooth enamel Parotiditis Calluses on the dorsal surface of the hands Electrolyte imbalance Often normal body weight (may be slightly overweight)
What is the cause of erosion of the tooth enamel?	Repeated exposure to gastric acid secondary to induced vomiting
What is parotiditis?	Swelling or infection of the parotid glands, usually secondary to vomiting
What causes the development of calluses on the back of the hands?	Scraping fingers along teeth while inducing vomiting
What is a very serious consequence of the repeated induced vomiting seen in bulimia nervosa?	Esophageal varices and/or Mallory-Weiss tears from repeated retching
What is the prominent psychological element of bulimia nervosa?	Secretive binge eating followed by purging
How can purging be accomplished?	Induced vomiting Laxative/diuretic/enema use Excessive exercise
What are some of the psychosocial features of patients with bulimia?	Poor self-image Depression and other mood disorders
What is the best treatment for bulimia nervosa?	Psychotherapy Behavior therapy Antidepressants—selective serotonin reuptake inhibitors (SSRIs) preferred Nutrition education Regular meals Healthy exercise

CHAPTER 18

Neuropsychiatric Disorders in Childhood

PERVASIVE DEVELOPMENT DISORDERS

What are the primary characteristics of the pervasive development disorders?	Failure to acquire or early loss of communication and social interaction skills
What are the pervasive development disorders?	Autistic disorder Asperger's disorder Rett's disorder Childhood disintegrative disorder
Which disorder is characterized by significant communication problems, difficulty in forming social relationships, repetitive behavior, and unusual abilities?	Autistic disorder
What term describes the unusual abilities (e.g., memory; calculation skills) that some autistic patients have?	Savant
The onset of autistic disorder must be before what age?	3 years of age
What is the risk of autism in monozygotic twins and siblings?	Increased risk due to genetic component
The incidence of autistic disorder is increased in which conditions?	Congenital anomalies Perinatal complications Congenital rubella

	Phenylketonuria Fragile X syndrome Tuberous sclerosis
Which brain abnormalities are associated with autism?	Seizures Electroencephalogram (EEG) abnormalities Anatomic and function abnormalities
Which gender is most likely to be affected by autism?	Males; 4× more likely
Which gender is more severely affected with mental retardation in autism?	Females
How is autistic disorder treated?	Psychotherapy aimed at increasing communication, social, and self-care skills
What is the IQ of many autistic patients?	Generally low; may have normal nonverbal IQ
Which disorder is a milder form of autism?	Asperger's disorder
What are the primary deficits in a patient with Asperger's?	Problems forming social relationships Repetitive behavior Acute interest in obscure topics
Which areas of functioning are normal in Asperger's but are usually deficient in autistic patients?	Cognitive and verbal skills
Which disorder is characterized by a decrease in social, verbal, and cognitive development after a period of normal functioning?	Rett's disorder
What are the primary characteristics of Rett's disorder?	Stereotyped hand-wringing movements Poor coordination Impaired language development Loss of hand skills Loss of social engagement Deceleration of head growth
Which gender is primarily affected by Rett's disorder?	Females
What happens to males affected by Rett's disorder?	Die before birth

What is the genetic inheritance of Rett's disorder?
X-linked

Which rare disorder is characterized by a diminution of cognitive, motor, social, and verbal development after 2 to 10 years of normal functioning?
Childhood disintegrative disorder

Which gender has the highest incidence of childhood disintegrative disorder?
Boys

DISRUPTIVE BEHAVIOR DISORDERS

What are the primary characteristics of disruptive behavior disorders?
Improper behavior; problems with school performance and social relationships

Which disorders are classified as disruptive behavior disorders?
Conduct disorder
Oppositional defiant disorder

Which disorder is characterized by insistent behavior that violates social norms, deviation from societal and parental rules, property destruction, and aggressive behavior?
Conduct disorder

What are examples of the behaviors that violate social norms that are common in patients with conduct disorder?
Arson
Theft
Animal harm
Assault

If a person is 18 years or older and exhibits the symptoms of conduct disorder, which disorder do they likely have?
Antisocial personality disorder

Which disorder is characterized by persistent disobedient, defiant, and negative behavior toward figures in authority?
Oppositional defiant disorder

What is the significant difference between oppositional defiant disorder and conduct disorder?
Persons with oppositional defiant disorder are not likely to violate social norms or harm people/property.

What are the primary treatment modalities for the disruptive behavior disorders?
Psychotherapy structured environment

ATTENTION DEFICIT HYPERACTIVITY DISORDER

What are the primary characteristics of attention deficit hyperactivity disorder (ADHD)?	Inattention Hyperactivity Impulsivity Impairment in multiple settings
Which gender is most likely to be affected by ADHD?	Boys are most likely to be affected
By definition, ADHD symptoms must be evident by which age to be given the classification of ADHD?	Before 7 years of age
How long must the symptoms of ADHD be present to be given the classification of ADHD?	At least 6 months
What percentage of the general child population in the United States is affected by ADHD?	3% to 7%
What is the intelligence level of persons with ADHD?	Normal intelligence
What percentage of ADHD patients have symptoms that persist into adulthood?	20%
What are the primary treatment modalities of ADHD?	Stimulants—usually amphetamines
What is a new medication that has been prescribed for individuals with ADHD over the age of 6?	Atomoxetine (a non-stimulant medication)
Which single drug is most widely prescribed for ADHD?	Methylphenidate

OTHER NEUROPSYCHIATRIC DISORDERS OF CHILDHOOD

Which disorder is characterized by chronic motor and vocal tics and involuntary use of profanity?	Tourette disorder
In which age group is Tourette disorder most likely to be diagnosed?	Usually 7 to 8 years of age; onset usually by 21 years of age
Tourette disorder has a genetic relationship to which two psychiatric disorders?	ADHD Obsessive-compulsive disorder

What is the primary treatment for Tourette disorder?	Antipsychotics (such as haloperidol or risperidone)
Which disorder is characterized by excessive and inappropriate anxiety concerning separation from parents, caretakers, and their home and production of physical complaints to avoid going to school?	Separation anxiety disorder
What is the most common age of onset in a person who presents with separation anxiety disorder?	7 to 8 years of age
Which treatment modalities are most effective in the treatment of separation anxiety disorder?	Psychotherapy, especially cognitive behavioral therapy
Which disorder is characterized by a refusal to verbally communicate in some or all social situations in which the child may communicate with gestures?	Selective mutism
In which gender is selective mutism more common?	Girls
Selective mutism has a poor prognosis if it persists after which age?	10 years of age
What is the primary trigger for the onset of separation anxiety disorder and selective mutism?	Stressful life events
What is the most common treatment modality for selective mutism?	Family and behavioral therapy

CHAPTER 19

Suicide: Epidemiology and Risk Factors

SUICIDE

What is important to keep in mind when approaching the topic of suicide on the United States Medical Licensing Exam (USMLE) Step 1?

There is only a limited amount of information that you will be asked about regarding suicide. Always think *safety* first when given a question regarding a psychiatric disorder. Statistics, demographics, and risk factors, and comorbid medical disorders will probably be the focus of the exam content. Many of the questions will come in the form of a case scenario written to ascertain if you know the correlation between suicide and comorbid mental health diagnoses such as depression, bipolar disorder, and/or chemical dependence.

What is the national rate of suicide in the United States?

As of 2002, suicide ranks tenth as the leading cause of death.

Who is most at risk of committing suicide?

A White male over 65 years with comorbid depression and/or an alcoholic who has suffered a loss or endured some type of stressor (physical, social, or professional). Having a medical illness, having the perception of a serious medical illness, and taking three or more prescription medications puts a patient at risk, as well.

Who commits suicide more, men or women?

1. Remember, in every age group, men commit suicide three times more than women in the United States and Europe. However, women attempt suicide four times as much.
2. In Asia and some Latin American countries, adolescent males and females have comparable suicide rates.

What age group has the highest suicide rate?

1. The elderly (65 and older). Despite composing only 14% of the population, they comprise about 18% to 25% of the total suicide percentage.
2. The elderly suicide rate is 40 per 100,000 persons in comparison to the national U.S. rate of 12 per 100,000.

What has happened to the suicide rate in child and adolescent groups over the last 40 years?

It has risen significantly over the last 40 years with a mortality rate of 12%.

What is the most significant risk factor of suicide?

A previous attempt.
You should become extremely cautious if the attempt was recent (e.g., within 3 months of the current time frame and if the nature of the attempt was well-thought out and deliberate).

What are other risk factors for suicide (in decreasing order)?

Persons over 45

Alcohol dependence

History of violence or aggression

Male gender

How is suicide committed or attempted?

Historically, men tend to use more violent methods such as shooting or hanging whereas women more often attempt by overdosing or drowning. As of 2000, the number one method of suicide for both genders is firearms.

Is there racial disparity among those who commit suicide?

Yes, it remains that Whites commit suicide more than any ethnic, minority group for all age groups. (However, the suicide rate among Black males is slowly increasing.)

What are the most common comorbid medical disorders associated with suicide?

1. Major depression—the order of the most common comorbid psychiatric diagnoses is major depression > alcohol dependence > depressive disorder unspecified > schizophrenia > any Axis II diagnoses > and lastly bipolar disorder.
2. Substance use, abuse, and dependence on illicit drugs are also commonly comorbid with suicide. Psychotic symptoms associated with depression, schizophrenia, or substance use is also a risk factor for suicide.

At what stage, in major depression, is suicide attempted?

1. For adults, suicide is most attempted after pharmacologic treatment has begun. The patient has more energy and is better able to function but low mood and hopelessness may persist.
2. There is not a high likelihood that a question about children and suicide will be asked since the Food and Drug Administration (FDA) black box warning of increased risk of suicidal ideation in children who are beginning antidepressant medication is newly mandated. However, be conservative in your management if you are given this question. You always want to employ a multidisciplinary team approach including family, behavioral, and occupational therapy regardless of whether medications are prescribed to a child. You will always be safe if you choose psycho education of parents and the child. Remember, under the new FDA rules, any child on an antidepressant must be seen once a week by a psychiatrist or physician for the first month and every other week for the next 2 months.

When do you assess for suicidality?

At every follow-up

1. Ideation
2. Plan (possibility and practicality)
3. Intent to carry out the plan (e.g.,"I would shoot myself if I had a gun" vs. "I will shoot myself with the loaded gun in the bedroom closet.")

Can suicide attempts be predicted?

No. There is no predictive or diagnostic test. Clinical studies have found a lower amount of the serotonin metabolite, 5-hydroxyindoleacetic acid (5-HIAA), in the cerebral spinal fluid in some persons who commit suicide. However, there are no confirmatory, causal links that have been made.

Can suicidal ideation be treated?

There is no treatment per se. First—think of the patient's safety. If there are mental health and social supports in place, one can consider discharging a patient who comes to the emergency room—*only if there is not a suicide plan or intent*. However, if suicidal ideation coexists with a plan and/or intent, go with hospitalization. Involuntary commitment to an inpatient psychiatric hospital may be necessary. Be conservative and protective with your efforts.

What is the primary goal in treating a patient with suicidal ideation?

The goal is to reduce the psychiatric symptoms and address the psychological and/or chemical dependence issues that are causing the suicidal ideation.

What are protective factors from suicide?

1. Marriage. Single persons that are divorced, have never married, or widowed have higher suicide rates than married persons. Living alone and limited social and family support are also risk factors.
2. Employment. Persons who are unemployed have higher suicide rates. However, among employed U.S. citizens, those working in professional roles (doctors, lawyers, and in law enforcement) have higher suicide rates than nonprofessional persons.

3. No family history of a completed suicide or an attempted suicide is protective because once suicide occurs, it seemingly decreases the social 'taboo' of suicide in the family.

Does religion impact suicide rates?

Yes, persons belonging to Jewish and Catholic faiths have lower suicide rates than Protestants.

CHAPTER 20

Psychological Testing

PSYCHOLOGICAL TESTS

What five parameters do psychological tests assess?

Achievement
Intelligence
Depression
Personality
Neuropsychologic
Functioning

What are the two types of tests utilized in psychological testing?

Objective
Projective

Which type of test is based on questions that include true-false, fill-in-the-blank, matching, and multiple choice questions and are based on questions that are scored easily? These tests are easier to analyze statistically.

Objective tests

Which type of test is used to determine a person's conflicts, motives, perceptions, and thoughts on the basis of the person's interpretations of questions? In these tests, there are no right or wrong answers.

Projective tests

What factors can influence performance on psychological testing?

Cultural and/or language barriers
Anxiety
Motivation
Educational differences

Achievement Tests

What are achievement tests used for?

To determine an individual's mastery of a particular subset of instructional material

Which test is designed to measure reading recognition, spelling, and arithmetic computation?	Wide Range Achievement Test
Which achievement test is commonly used to evaluate students at various grade levels in the areas of vocabulary, mathematics, spelling, social studies, word study skills, reading comprehension, listening, and language?	Stanford achievement test
What are names of other popular achievement tests?	Iowa SAT GMAT GRE MCAT USMLE

Intelligence Tests

Which term is used to describe the ability to learn, understand, or to deal with new or trying situations?	Intelligence
Which term did Binet use to describe the average intellectual age of people with a specific chronological age?	Mental age
Which scale is used to determine a person's IQ?	Stanford-Binet scale
How is the IQ calculated?	Mental age/chronological age × 100
If a person has an IQ of 100, what does that indicate?	Mental and chronological age is equivalent
If a person has an IQ < 70, what does that indicate?	Mental retardation
What is the highest chronological age used to determine IQ?	15 years of age
What happens to the IQ throughout the course of a person's life?	Remains generally stable
Which IQ range indicates that a person has an average intelligence?	90 to 109
Which IQ range indicates borderline to low average intelligence?	71 to 89

Which IQ range indicates mild mental retardation?	50 to 70
Which IQ range indicates moderate mental retardation?	35 to 55
Which IQ range indicates severe mental retardation?	20 to 40
Which IQ range indicates profound mental retardation?	< 20
What is the genetic association with IQ in monozygotic twins?	Strong genetic component with an 85% concordance rate in monozygotic twins
How can substandard nutrition and illness affect IQ?	Negatively affects IQ
Which test is the most commonly used intelligence test?	Wechsler Adult Intelligence Scale-Revised (WAIS-R)
The Wechsler Adult Intelligence Scale-Revised has 11 subtests that evaluate which areas?	Verbal (six subtests) Performance (five subtests)
Which age group does the Wechsler Scale for Children-Revised (WISC-R) test?	6 to 16.5 years
Which age group does the Wechsler Preschool and Primary Scale of Intelligence (WPPSI) test?	4 to 6.5 years

Depression Tests

Which test is a patient-rated 21-itemscale that assesses the intensity of depression in individuals and is the most widely used test to assess depression?	Beck Depression Inventory
Which test is a physician-rated 17-item scale that evaluates depressed mood, vegetative, and cognitive symptoms of depression, and comorbid anxiety symptoms?	Hamilton Depression Rating Scale
Which test is a 20-item scale in which an individual reports symptoms and their severity?	Zung Self-Rating Depression Scale

Which test is used as a global rating of depression severity that explores the extent to which an individual demonstrates depression based on verbal self-report, behavior, and secondary symptoms of depression?

Raskin Depression Scale

Personality Tests

What are personality tests used to measure?

Personality characteristics

Defense mechanisms

Psychopathology

Emotions

Conflicts

Which personality test is a true-false test designed to assess a number of major patterns of personality, emotional, and behavioral disorders?

Minnesota Multiphasic Personality Inventory

Which personality test utilizes picture cards to stimulate stories or descriptions about relationships or social situations and can help identify dominant drives, emotions, sentiments, conflicts, and complexes?

Thematic Apperception Test

Which personality test utilizes inkblots to determine what a person perceives in enigmatic and highly ambiguous shapes?

Rorschach Test

Which personality test asks the patient to complete short sentences started by the examiner?

Sentence Completion Test

Which of the personality tests is an objective test?

Minnesota Multiphasic Personality Inventory

Neuropsychological Tests

Which parameters are neuropsychological tests used to measure?

Memory

Intelligence

Reasoning

Attention

Language function

Concentration

On what type of patients are neuropsychological tests used?
Patients with neurological problems (e.g., brain damage, dementia)

Which neuropsychological test is used to detect and localize brain lesions and determine their effects?
Halstead-Reitan Battery

Which neuropsychological test is used to identify specific types of brain dysfunction and right or left cerebral dominance?
Luria-Nebraska Neuropsychological Battery

Which neuropsychological test is a brief test of visual-motor integration that may provide interpretive information about an individual's development and psychological functioning?
Bender Visual Motor Gestalt test

PSYCHOLOGICAL AND BIOLOGICAL EVALUATION

Which test is utilized to determine a patient's current state of mental functioning?
Mental Status Examination

Which test suppresses the secretion of cortisol in an individual with a normal hypothalamic-pituitary axis but shows limited or absent suppression in patients with major depressive disorder?
Dexamethasone Suppression Test

If a psychiatric patient presents with limited or absent suppression of cortisol, which two treatment methods may be helpful?
Electroconvulsive therapy
Antidepressants

In which other psychiatric conditions may one see a limited or absent suppression of cortisol?
Schizophrenia
Dementia
Anorexia nervosa

Which test is the initial test used to determine if there is an endocrine dysfunction in persons who present with psychiatric issues?
Thyroid function tests

Hyperthyroidism may mimic which psychiatric condition?
Anxiety

Hypothyroidism may mimic which psychiatric condition?
Depression

In which other endocrine disorders might psychiatric symptoms present?	Addison's disease Cushing's syndrome
Which test measures electrical current within the brain?	Electroencephalogram (EEG)
Which condition(s) does an EEG identify?	Delirium Demyelinating illness Epilepsy
Which test measures electrical activity in the brain in response to sensory stimulation?	Evoked potentials
Which condition(s) do evoked potentials identify?	Brain responses in a coma Hearing and vision loss in infants
Which substance is used to relax patients during an interview?	Sodium amobarbital
Which condition(s) can a sodium amobarbital interview identify?	Conversion disorder Dissociative disorder
Which test measures the electrical resistance of the skin and interprets it as an image of activity in certain parts of the body?	Galvanic skin response
What condition(s) does a galvanic skin response measure?	Stress
Administration of which two substances evokes panic attacks in susceptible patients?	CO_2 inhalation Sodium lactate administration
Which tests are used to identify biochemical conditions, anatomy of neural tissues, and brain activity during specific tasks?	Neuroimaging (computerized axial tomography [CAT], magnetic resonance imaging [MRI], magnetic resonance angiography [MRA], and positron emission tomography [PET] scans)

CHAPTER 21

Sexuality

SEXUAL DEVELOPMENT

Which gender is the default pattern for sexual development?	Female
Gonad differentiation is dependent upon the presence of which chromosome?	Y chromosome
Which gene present on the Y chromosome influences gonad development?	Testis-determining factor
Which duct system present in male embryos helps form genitalia?	Wolffian duct system
Which duct system in female embryos help form female genitalia?	Mullerian duct system
Which organ secretes hormones that direct the differentiation of male internal and external genitalia?	Testes
How does exposure to different levels of hormones during prenatal life influence humans?	It causes gender differences in certain areas of the brain.
What term(s) describe an individual's sense of being male or female?	Gender identity
At which age(s) does gender awareness become evident?	2 or 3 years of age
What term(s) describes the expression of gender identity in society?	Gender role
What term(s) describes the conflict people experience when they feel as if they were born as the wrong gender?	Gender identity disorder, which is also called transsexuality
Which term(s) describe a preference for members of the opposite sex (heterosexuality) or preference for members of the same sex (homosexuality)?	Sexual orientation

According to the Diagnostic and Statistical Manual of Mental Disorders—Fourth Edition (DSM-IV), is homosexuality a dysfunction of sexual expression?
No, it is a normal variant.

Which gender has the highest prevalence of homosexuality?
Males with 3% to 10% prevalence compared with a 1% to 5% prevalence in females.

What type of behavior in childhood may be predictive of later homosexual orientation?
Cross-gender behavior → stronger correlation in males

Which hormones have been shown to influence sexual orientation?
Prenatal hormones → low levels of androgens in males and high levels of androgens in females

Which evidence has been reported, which indicates that genetics plays a role in homosexuality?
Higher concordance rate in monozygotic twins than in dizygotic twins

On which chromosome have genetic markers been found in homosexuals?
X chromosome

What type of psychological treatment is commonly used to treat homosexuality?
None. Since homosexuality is not a dysfunction, no psychological treatment is necessary.

SEXUAL DEVELOPMENT AND PHYSIOLOGIC ABNORMALITIES

Which disorder is characterized by body cells that are not responsive to androgens and testicles that may appear as inguinal or labial masses?
Androgen insensitivity which is also called testicular feminization

What is the genotype of a person with androgen insensitivity?
XY

What is the phenotype of a person with androgen insensitivity?
Female

Which disorder is characterized by an adrenal gland that is unable to produce the proper amount of cortisol which leads to a significantly increased androgen secretion?
Congenital adrenal hyperplasia which is also called adrenogenital syndrome

What is the genotype of a person with congenital adrenal hyperplasia?
XX

What is the phenotype of a person with congenital adrenal hyperplasia?
Female with genitalia that are masculine

What is the sexual orientation of 33% of patients with congenital adrenal hyperplasia?

Lesbian

Which disorder is characterized by a short stature, webbed neck, and streak ovaries?

Turner's syndrome

What is the genotype of a person with Turner's syndrome?

XO

What is the phenotype of a person with Turner's syndrome?

Female

HORMONES AND THEIR INFLUENCE ON BEHAVIOR

Which hormone may be decreased by an increase in stress?

Testosterone

Which three hormones commonly used in medical treatment of conditions such as prostate cancer decrease androgen production and in turn reduces sexual interest and behavior?

Androgen antagonists

Estrogens

Progesterone

What happens to a woman's sex drive when she reaches menopause and ages?

Nothing. Since estrogen is minimally involved in libido, there is no reduction in sex drive.

Which hormone is believed to play the most important role in sex drive in both genders?

Testosterone

Which hormone may decrease sexual behavior and interest in women?

Progesterone → this hormone is in many oral contraceptives.

SEXUAL RESPONSE CYCLE

What are the four stages in the sexual response cycle developed by Masters and Johnson?

Excitement

Plateau

Orgasm

Resolution

What is the primary characteristic of the excitement stage in men?

Penile erection

What are characteristics of the excitement stage in women?

Clitoral erection

Vaginal lubrication

Labial swelling

Uterus raises in pelvic cavity → tenting effect

What characteristics of the excitement stage are common to men and women?	Nipple erection Elevation of blood pressure, pulse, and respiration
What are characteristics of the plateau stage in men?	Increased upward movement and size of testes Secretion of drops of sperm-containing fluid
What is the primary characteristic of the plateau stage in women?	Muscular contraction of the outer one-third of the vagina which forms the orgasmic platform
What characteristics of the plateau stage are common to both men and women?	Chest and face flushing Greater elevation of blood pressure, pulse, and respiration
What is the primary characteristic of the orgasm stage in men?	Ejaculation of seminal fluid
What is the primary characteristic of the orgasm stage in women?	Muscular contractions of the uterus and vagina
What is the characteristic of the orgasm stage that is common to both men and women?	Muscular contractions of the anal sphincter
What are characteristics of the recovery stage in men?	Refractory period in which stimulation is not possible
What happens to the refractory period of men as they age?	Increases
What is the primary characteristic of the recovery stage in women?	Minimal or no refractory period
What are characteristics of the refractory period that are common to both men and women?	Physiological systems return to their prestimulated states (e.g., cardiovascular, respiratory) Muscle relaxation

SEXUAL DYSFUNCTION

Which term(s) describe problems in stages of the sexual response cycle?	Sexual dysfunction
Which disorder is characterized by pain associated with sexual intercourse?	Dyspareunia
Which gender is most likely to experience dyspareunia?	Females

Which disorder is characterized by inability to maintain vaginal lubrication throughout the duration of a sexual act?	Female sexual arousal disorder → occurs in approximately 20% of women
Which disorder is characterized by decreased interest in sexual activity?	Hypoactive sexual desire
Which disorder is characterized by problems with maintaining erections?	Male erectile disorder also called impotence
What are the three types of male erectile disorder?	Primary Secondary Situational
What are characteristics of primary male erectile disorder?	Never has the ability to achieve an erection sufficient for penetration → this is a rare lifelong disorder
What are characteristics of secondary male erectile disorder?	A current inability to achieve erections despite previous success → this is an acquired disorder
What are characteristics of situational male erectile disorder?	Difficulty in maintaining erection in some situations
Which disorder is characterized by an inability to achieve an orgasm?	Orgasmic disorder → this disorder can be lifelong or acquired
Which disorder is characterized by anxiety and ejaculation before a man desires?	Premature ejaculation
Which stage of the sexual response cycle is affected by premature ejaculation?	Plateau phase → absent or reduced
Which disorder is characterized by avoidance or aversion to sexual activity?	Sexual aversion disorder
Which disorder is characterized by painful muscular spasms in the outer one-third of the vagina making pelvic examination or sexual intercourse difficult?	Vaginismus
Which behavioral treatment stimulates a person's senses during sexual activity to reduce the pressure one experiences when trying to achieve an erection or orgasm?	Sensate-focus exercise
Which behavioral technique helps a man to identify the stage before emission so that his partner can exert pressure on the coronal ridge on the glans penis bilaterally to reduce erection?	Squeeze technique

What is the primary goal of the squeeze technique?	To treat premature ejaculation
Which segment of the nervous system is used to initiate an erection?	Parasympathetic
Which segment of the nervous system is used to initiate an ejaculation?	Sympathetic
Which behavioral technique(s) are used to reduce anxiety associated with sexual performance?	Hypnosis Relaxation techniques Systematic desensitization
Which sexual stimuli might a physician recommend to determine what is most effective for an individual?	Masturbation
Which drug is used to treat erectile dysfunction by blocking the phosphodiester-5 (PDE-5) enzyme thereby inhibiting cyclic guanosine monophosphate (cGMP)?	Sildenafil citrate (Viagra)
What is the role of cGMP in sexual stimulation of the penis?	It is a vasodilator which allows an erection to persist.
Which drug is used to increase the availability of dopamine in the brain in patients with erectile disorder and female arousal disorder?	Apomorphine (Uprima)
What injection method is used to treat erectile dysfunction?	Intracorporeal injection of vasodilators
Which vasodilators are commonly injected in intracorporeal injection?	Papaverine Phentolamine

PARAPHILIAS

What term describes the use of unusual objects of sexual desire or unusual sexual activities?	Paraphilia
Which paraphilia is most common and is characterized by a person who achieves sexual gratification from children <14 years of age?	Pedophilia → perpetrator must be at least 16 years of age and at least 5 years older than victim
Which paraphilia is characterized by exposing genitals to strangers?	Exhibitionism

Which paraphilia is characterized by achieving sexual gratification from inanimate objects?
Fetishism

Which paraphilia is characterized by recurrent urges to rub against or touch a noncompliant person in a sexual manner?
Frotteurism

Which paraphilia is characterized by a sexual gratification with corpses?
Necrophilia

Which paraphilia is characterized by causing humiliation and physical suffering to achieve sexual gratification?
Sexual sadism

Which paraphilia is characterized by being the recipient of humiliation and physical suffering to achieve sexual gratification?
Sexual masochism

Which paraphilia is characterized by achieving sexual gratification by wearing women's clothing?
Transvestic fetishism

Which paraphilia is characterized by watching others engage in sexual activity and undress?
Voyeurism

INFLUENCE OF MEDICAL CONDITIONS ON SEXUALITY

What effect does a myocardial infarction have on sexual activity?
Decreased libido
Erectile dysfunction

Which postmyocardial infarction patients can resume sexual activity?
Patients who can tolerate increases in heart rate from 110 to 130 bpm

Which problem is common in diabetic men?
Erectile dysfunction

What are the two main causes of erectile dysfunction in diabetics?
Diabetic neuropathy
Vascular changes

What is the primary treatment for erectile dysfunction in diabetics?
Metabolic control monitored by Hemoglobin A_{1c} level

What effect does spinal cord dysfunction have on sexual functioning in men?
Decreased fertility
Erectile dysfunction
Orgasmic dysfunction
Reduced testosterone levels
Retrograde ejaculation into the bladder

What effect does pregnancy have on sexual functioning?	Decreased sex drive → most common Increased sex drive and pelvic vasocongestion may occur
During what time period prior to pregnancy should a woman cease sexual activity?	4 weeks before expected delivery

EFFECTS OF DRUGS AND NEUROTRANSMITTERS ON SEXUALITY

Decreased **availability of which neurotransmitter(s) causes a** ***decrease*** **in erection?**	Dopamine (e.g., chlorpromazine, haloperidol) Norepinephrine β (e.g., propranolol, metoprolol)
Increased **availability of which neurotransmitter(s) causes a** ***decrease*** **in ejaculation and orgasm?**	Serotonin (e.g., fluoxetine, sertraline, trazodone)
Increased **availability of which neurotransmitter(s) causes an** ***increase*** **in erection?**	Dopamine (e.g., levodopa) Norepinephrine in α_2 in the periphery (e.g., yohimbine)
Which drug(s) of abuse causes increased libido with ***acute use*****?**	Alcohol Marijuana
Which drug(s) of abuse causes increased libido?	Amphetamines Cocaine
Which drug(s) of abuse causes erectile dysfunction due to increased estrogen availability as a result of liver damage?	Alcohol → with *chronic use*
Which drugs(s) of abuse causes reduced testosterone levels in men and lowered pituitary gonadotropin levels in women?	Marijuana → with *chronic use*
Which drug(s) of abuse causes reduced libido and inhibited ejaculation?	Heroin Methadone

CHAPTER 22

Abuse and Aggression

CHILDREN AND ELDER ABUSE AND NEGLECT

What are the primary types of child and elder abuse?

Physical

Sexual

Emotional

What are the primary traits of a child abuser?

Low socioeconomic status

Social isolation

Substance abuse

Close relationship to abused (e.g., father, mother)

History of victimization by spouse or caretaker

Which gender is most likely to be the perpetrator of child abuse?

Female

What are the primary traits of a child that experiences child abuse?

Mild physical impairment

Low birth weight, premature infant

Child that is perceived as mentally slow or different

"Fussy" or "colicky" infant

Hyperactive

What is the most common age range of children that are abused?

<5 years of age

What are key signs of child neglect?

Lack of proper nutrition

Poor personal hygiene

What are common sites of bruises on a victim of child abuse?

Lower back and buttocks → areas not commonly injured during normal activities

What type of marks might one see on a victim of child abuse?

Belt and belt buckle marks

What are characteristics of the fractures on a victim of child abuse?	Fractures at different stages of healing Spiral fractures → due to twisting limbs
What are the two primary burn types on victims of child abuse?	Cigarette burns Immersion burns on legs, feet, or buttocks → child is immersed in scalding water
What are the primary traits of an elder abuser?	Low socioeconomic status Social isolation Substance abuse Close relationship to abused (e.g., spouse, offspring) → person with whom the elder lives and receives financial support from
What are the primary traits of an elder who experiences elder abuse?	Some decline of mental functioning (e.g., dementia) Economical or physical dependence on others Not likely to report injuries as abuse → will state that they injured themselves
What are key signs of elder neglect?	Lack of proper nutrition Poor personal hygiene Lack of proper medication or health aids (e.g., prescription drugs, dentures, cane)
What are characteristics of the bruises seen on a victim of elder abuse?	Bilateral arm bruises from being grabbed
What is the annual incidence of child sexual abuse cases in the United States?	More than 250,000 cases
Has the likelihood of reporting child sexual abuse increased or decreased when compared with the past?	Increased
Which gender is more likely to report sexual abuse during their lifetime?	Girls → 25% will report vs. 12% boys
Which gender is most likely to be the perpetrator of child sexual abuse?	Males
Will the perpetrator of a child sexual abuse more likely be an acquaintance or stranger?	Acquaintance (e.g., father, uncle, mother, and so forth)

What are some traits of child sexual abusers?

Interpersonal relationship problems (e.g., marriage problems)

History of substance abuse

May have a history of pedophilia

What is the primary age range of children who are victims of sexual abuse?

9 to 12 years of age

What emotions is the victim of a child sexual abuse likely to experience?

Guilt

Shame

Fear of abuser's response if he or she notified someone else of his or her experience

What are the common physical signs of child sexual abuse?

Sexually transmitted infection (e.g., human papillomavirus [HPV], herpes, chlamydia)

Recurrent urinary tract infection (UTI)

Genital or anal injury

Note: Physical signs may be absent in a victim of child sexual abuse.

What are common psychological signs of child sexual abuse?

Inappropriate knowledge about sexual events out of proportion for a given age range

Excessive initiation of sexual activity with peers

What are common physical signs of elder sexual abuse?

Genital bruising

Vaginal bleeding in women

What types of emotional abuse do children experience?

Lack of caregiver attention and love

Physical neglect

Caregiver rejection

What types of emotion abuse do elders experience?

Neglect of needed care (e.g., medical, hygiene, and so forth.)

Economic exploitation

How many cases of child and elder abuse are reported annually?

1,000,000 cases each

What is the physician's responsibility if he or she suspects child or elder abuse?

Physician *must* report the case to appropriate social service agency

DOMESTIC PARTNER ABUSE

What are primary findings seen in women who are victims of domestic violence?

Broken bones

Bruises

Blackened eyes

What factor can greatly increase the likelihood of an abused person being killed by his or her abuser?

If the abused person leaves the abuser

What is the primary gender of the perpetrator of domestic violence?

Male

What are the characteristics of the abuser in a domestic violence situation?

Substance abuse

Bad temper

Angry

Threatens to kill the abused

Apologetic after abuse has occurred

What are the characteristics of the abused in a domestic violence situation?

May be pregnant

May not report abuse to police

May not leave the abuser

Blame themselves for the abuse

Emotional and financial dependence on abuser

What characteristic is common to both the abused and the abuser in a domestic violence situation?

Low self-esteem

What is the role of the physician, in terms of reporting, if notified of domestic violence abuse?

The physician does not have mandatory reporting since the abused is generally a competent adult. The physician can provide emotional support and encourage the abused to report the violence.

SEXUAL VIOLENCE

What is the definition of sexual assault?

A person commits a *sexual* assault when he or she uses *force* or the threat of *force* to touch another person *sexually* in a way that person does not want or when that person cannot give *consent* because of physical or mental inability. **Note:** Sexual assault is the legal term for rape.

What are examples of force that can be used to commit a sexual assault?	Manipulation Coercion Physical force Use of weapons Use of isolation Use of substances —alcohol and other drugs
What is the definition of consent?	Giving permission by giving a "yes" response
What is the reason why a perpetrator commits a sexual assault?	To gain power. This is not a crime about sex. Sex is the tool used to gain power over an individual.
What term describes oral and anal penetration?	Sodomy
What is the primary age group of a rapist?	<25 years of age
What is the racial background of a perpetrator of sexual assault?	Perpetrator will generally be the same race as the victim
Which substance is most frequently used in cases of sexual assault?	Alcohol
What percentage of rapes are acquaintance rapes (i.e., the victim knows the perpetrator)?	Approximately 85% of rapes
What percentage of rapes is reported to the police?	Approximately 10%—rape is the most underreported violent crime in the United States.
What is the age group most likely to experience a sexual assault?	16 to 24 years of age
What is the most common place for a sexual assault to occur?	In the victim's home
Who do people generally blame as the reason for a sexual assault to occur?	The victim (e.g., wearing tight clothing, drinking too much alcohol)
Which disorder do/may sexual assault survivors experience?	Posttraumatic stress disorder
Which type of treatment is the best option for survivors of sexual assault?	Group therapy
Is it possible for spouses to be convicted of committing a sexual assault against each other?	Yes
What terms describes consensual sex that is considered rape?	Statutory rape

With which group(s) of people would consensual sex be considered statutory rape?

People < 16 or 18 years of age depending upon the state

Disabled persons

What is the role of the physician if they suspect a sexual assault?

The physician does not have mandatory reporting since the abused is generally a competent adult. The physician can provide emotional support and encourage the abused to report the violence.

AGGRESSION

What is happening to the incidence of homicide in the United States?

Decreasing

Which socioeconomic group is most likely to be affected by a homicide?

Low socioeconomic groups

Which weapon is most commonly used in a homicide?

Guns

What traits found in children are good predictors of their likelihood to become violent adults?

High levels of aggression and antisocial behavior

Victim of physical and sexual abuse

Cruelty to animals

Low IQ

How does violence on television or video games influence aggression in children?

Direct correlation with increased aggression in children

Which gender is most likely to be most aggressive?

Males

Why are males the most aggressive gender?

They have a higher level of androgen

Why are many body builders and some professional athletes likely to show increased aggression?

Use of androgenic or anabolic steroids increases aggression

Use of which drugs is associated with increased aggression?

Alcohol

Amphetamines

Cocaine

Phencyclidine

Marijuana (high doses)

Which neurotransmitter(s) is associated with increased aggression?	Dopamine Norepinephrine
Which neurotransmitter(s) is associated with decreased aggression?	Serotonin γ-Aminobutyric acid (GABA)
What type of injury is most likely to be associated with violence?	Head injury

CHAPTER 23

Health-Care Provider—Patient Relationship

What is the importance of rapport?

It allows the physician to establish a relationship with the patient that contributes to the effectiveness of care. The patient needs to feel understood and accepted by a physician they respect.

What is compliance?

Compliance is the degree to which the patient follows the advice of the treating physician. The treatment plan may include medications, changes in lifestyle, social programs (AA), and returning for appointments.

What factors lead to increased patient compliance?

1. Good rapport (most important!)
2. Patient feeling ill (patients do not worry as much when they are asymptomatic)
3. Physician's attitude toward the treatment (do you believe in it?)
4. Patient's involvement in creating the treatment plan
5. Understandable, uncomplicated treatment plan (better if written out on paper too)
6. Frequent visits with less waiting room time
7. Good support structure

How might a physician make a treatment plan less complicated?

The treatment plan can be simplified by limiting:
1. The number of medications the patient is taking
2. The number of times the medications is taken per day
3. The number of changes made at each visit

Is compliance influenced by gender, age, race, income, IQ, education, or religion?

No. However, psychiatric patients are less compliant than medical patients.

Why are patients with psychiatric problems less likely to seek treatment?

Patients with psychiatric conditions are less likely to seek treatment due to the stigma associated with mental illness.

Do morbidity and mortality rates change for patients with psychiatric conditions?

Yes. Patients with psychiatric illnesses, particularly schizophrenia, have an increased risk of medical illnesses that are not treated because either:
1. The patients are less likely to seek medical care
2. The patients are less likely to comply with treatment
3. Many physicians do not treat these patients equally due to stigma

How should a physician deal with noncompliance?

1. Uncover the reasons behind the behavior
2. Establish a more suitable treatment
3. Suggest that a family member assist the patient

When should a physician refer the patient to another physician?

A physician should refer the patient to other physicians when the treatment necessary is outside his or her realm of training.

How should a physician respond to a patient who is speaking negatively about another physician?

1. Listen quietly
2. Suggest the patient to discuss these issues with the other physician.

Note: If there is anything particularly alarming occurring in the treatment, it should be further investigated.

Are all stressors negative?

No. Joyous events can be stressful as well as terrible ones, including getting married or moving to a new home. Increased stress of any kind has been shown to precipitate both physical and mental illnesses.

Which endocrinological system causes stressors to affect both physical and mental illness?

When stress is increased, the hypothalamic-pituitary adrenal (HPA) axis reacts by releasing adrenocorticotropic hormone (ACTH) and subsequently glucocorticoids which suppress the immune system. Chronic activation of this axis can lead to depression and anxiety.

What personality characteristics lead to increased morbidity and mortality related to heart disease?

Anger and hostility are correlated with increased risk for heart disease.

What interviewing technique elicits the least biased information from a patient?

Asking open-ended questions is generally the best way to obtain the initial information. It avoids influencing or "leading" the patient which can result in misdiagnosis and incorrect treatment. *Closed-ended questions* should be used *later in the interview to focus* in on specific problems.

At what point should a physician withhold information from a patient?

If the patient requests it.
Note: A family member may not make this decision for the patient unless the patient is a nonemancipated minor. However, a physician may advise the family that it is best to tell the minor the truth.

What is illness behavior?

Illness behavior has also been referred to as "the sick role" which describes how patients act or what they expect when they are sick (not going to work, being taken care of, going to the doctor). This behavior may be influenced by previous experiences and cultural views of illness.

What are the three immature defense mechanisms that patients use when they are diagnosed with a fatal illness?

Denial (first stage of Elizabeth Kubler Ross's stages of death and dying)

Regression (taking a childlike role)

Displacement (blame others, including the doctor)

How is pain classified?

Pain can be generated by *psychological* or *physical* factors that are either *acute* or *chronic*. In either circumstance, the physician must remember that the pain is experienced by the patient as "real."

What is the treatment plan for psychological pain?

1. Antidepressants (tricyclics and selective serotonin reuptake inhibitors [SSRIs])
2. Psychotherapy
3. Biofeedback
4. Hypnosis

What options can one utilize to treat physical pain?

1. Analgesics sometimes via different routes.
2. Nerve block
3. Radiation
4. Chemotherapy
5. Resection

Note: The treatment plan for physical pain will vary widely with the type of pain whether it be cancer pain, musculoskeletal, neurologic, and so forth.

How should pain medication be administered to patients suffering from chronic pain?

Give on a scheduled basis.
Note: Making the patient ask for pain medications when he or she needs it, puts him or her in a position that will ultimately make him or her appear "drug-seeking" to the nursing staff.

Which psychiatric disorders are most associated with pain disorder?

Depression and substance abuse

CHAPTER 24

Health Care in the United States

HEALTH STATUS AND DETERMINANTS

What is the percentage of physical illness that is due to individual patterns of living (e.g., lack of exercise, poor dietary choices, and smoking)?	Approximately 70%
What are the primary determinants of socioeconomic status?	Education level Income Occupation Residence
Which socioeconomic group tends to delay seeking health care and present with more progressive illnesses?	People of low socioeconomic status → due to lack of funds for health care
Which gender is most likely to seek medical care?	Female
Which gender has the lowest life expectancy?	Male
Which group of people has the lowest life expectancy with regards to race and gender?	Black males
Which group of people has the highest life expectancy with regards to race and gender?	Asian women
Which disease entities are women more likely to suffer from?	Acquired immunodeficiency syndrome (AIDS) → more likely to advance to AIDS when HIV+ (human immunodeficiency virus) Autoimmune diseases Illnesses linked to alcohol consumption Illnesses linked to cigarette smoking

Which group of people represents the fastest growing segment of the U.S. population?	Elderly
What is the percentage of health-care costs the elderly population is responsible for?	30%
Which ethnic minority represents the largest percent of the U.S. population?	Hispanic
What has happened to the birth rate of teenage girls over the last decade?	Declined → approximately 13%
What are the three leading causes of death in infants <1 year of age (rank in order from most common to least common)?	Congenital anomalies Sudden infant death syndrome (SIDS) Respiratory distress syndrome
What are the three leading causes of death in children between 1 and 4 years of age (rank in order from most common to least common)?	Accidents Congenital anomalies Cancer
What are the three leading causes of death in children between 5 and 14 years of age (rank in order from most common to least common)?	Accidents Cancer Homicide
What are the three leading causes of death in young adults between 15 and 24 years of age (rank in order from most common to least common)?	Accidents → mostly motor vehicle Homicide Suicide
What are the three leading causes of death in adults between 25 and 44 years of age (rank in order from most common to least common)?	Accidents HIV infections Cancer
What are the three leading causes of death in adults between 45 and 64 years of age (rank in order from most common to least common)?	Cancer Heart disease Stroke
What are the three leading causes of death in elderly over 65 years of age (rank in order from most common to least common)?	Heart disease Cancer Stroke
What is the leading cause of death in the United States, irrespective of age group?	Heart disease

In which race(s) is heart disease the leading cause of death?

Black

Native American

White

In which race(s) is cancer the leading cause of death?

Asian or Pacific Islander

HEALTH-CARE INSURANCE

What is the primary difference in health-care insurance coverage in the United States as compared to other industrialized countries?

The United States is the *only* industrialized country without publicly mandated government funded health care for *all* citizens.

How many people do not have health-care insurance?

Approximately 40 million people → approximately 16% of the U.S. population

Which economic group is most likely to be uninsured or underinsured?

People of the middle class under the age of 65 → since they do not qualify for government aid through programs such as Medicaid and Medicare

Which government program has been established to cover the health-care costs of the indigent population?

Medicaid

What coverage do patients with Medicaid receive?

Dialysis

Home health care

Hospice

Inpatient and outpatient hospital costs

Laboratory tests

Long-term nursing home care

Physician services

Prescription drugs

Which government program has been established to cover the health-care costs of the elderly population over the age of 65 years?

Medicare

In addition to the elderly population, what other segment of the population is covered by Medicare?

People with chronic disabilities and debilitating diseases

Note: These people can be from any age group.

What does Part A of Medicare cover?	Hospice care Inpatient hospital costs Nursing home care → maximum of 3 months coverage
What does Part B of Medicare cover?	Ambulance service Dialysis Laboratory tests Medical equipment Outpatient hospital care Physical therapy Physician bills Prescription drugs (limited) → e.g., immunosuppressive drugs and drugs used in nebulizers
Which part of Medicare is optional and requires a co-payment and deductible?	Part B → 20% co-payment and $100 deductible
What other options are available for assistance with prescription drugs for Medicare patients?	Medicare prescription drug plan—effective January 1, 2006. Insurance companies and other private companies will work with Medicare to offer these drug plans. They will negotiate discounts on drug prices.
What is used by Medicare to pay hospital bills?	Diagnosis-related groups (DRGs) → A certain amount is paid for cost of hospitalization for each illness instead of for the actual costs incurred
What two health-care costs are not covered by Medicare?	Long-term nursing care Outpatient prescription drugs
Which government-funded insurance plan is funded completely by the federal government?	Medicare. Medicaid receives funding from the federal and state governments both.
What are the primary sources of funding for health-care insurance for U.S. citizens?	Employee benefit People obtain health-care insurance on their own
Which not-for-profit insurance carrier provides insurance for 30% to 50% of working citizens in all 50 states?	Blue Cross/Blue Shield **Note:** Blue Cross covers hospital costs. Blue Shield covers diagnostic tests and physicians fees.

What are the two primary health plans offered by private health-care insurers?

Fee-for-service plans

Managed care plan

Which type of health-care insurance plan has high premiums and does not impose restrictions on provider choice?

Fee-for-service plans

What are the primary characteristics of a managed care plan?

Group of health-care providers are responsible for all aspects of an individual's health.

What are the primary characteristics of a health-care managed care plan?

Low premiums

Restrictions on provider choice

What are the types of health-care managed care plans?

Health maintenance organization (HMO)

Preferred provider organizations (PPOs)

Point of service (POS)

What is an HMO?

An HMO enters into contractual arrangements with health-care providers to form a "provider network." A contracted provider is one who provides services to health plan members at discounted rates in exchange for receiving health plan referrals. Members are required to see only providers within this network to have their healthcare paid for by the HMO. Members select a primary care physician (PCP), often called a "gatekeeper," who provides, arranges, coordinates, and authorizes all aspects of the member's health care.

What happens if the HMO member receives care outside of the network?

If the member receives care from a provider who isn't in the network, the HMO won't pay for care unless it was preauthorized by the HMO or deemed an emergency.

What are PPOs?

PPOs are similar to HMOs in that they enter into contractual arrangements with healthcare providers to form a "provider network." Unlike an HMO, members do not have a PCP (gatekeeper) nor do they have to use an in-network provider for their care. However, PPOs offer members "richer" benefits as financial incentives to use network providers.

What is a POS-managed care plan?

A POS plan is often called an HMO/PPO hybrid or an "open-ended" HMO. The reason it is called "point-of-service" is that members choose any option—HMO or PPO—each time they seek health care. Like an HMO and a PPO, a POS plan has a contracted provider network.

HEALTH-CARE COSTS

What are the health-care expenditures in the United States?

Approximately \$1.5 trillion → over 15% of the gross domestic product, the United State spends more on health care than any other industrialized country.

Which factors have contributed to the increase in health-care expenditures?

Larger percentage of elderly individuals

Medical technology advances

Medicaid and Medicare expenditures

What are the most expensive components of health care in the United States (rank items from most expensive to least expensive)?

1. Hospitalization
2. Physician costs
3. Nursing home costs
4. Prescription drugs
5. Medical supplies
6. Mental health services
7. Dental and other care

PHYSICIAN'S ROLE

How many physicians are there in the United States?

Approximately 700,000

What percentage of physicians are primary care physicians?

One-third of all physicians → this number is increasing, and it is projected that primary care physicians will account for nearly half of all physicians in the near future.

What is happening to the number of specialists in the United States?

It is decreasing

What is the average number of physician visits per year?

Five visits annually

Where do most physician-patient encounters occur for high socioeconomic status individuals?

Physician's office

Where do most physician-patient encounters occur for low socioeconomic status individuals?

Hospital emergency rooms

What are the two most common reasons that patients will seek medical attention?

Injuries

Upper respiratory ailments

HEALTH-CARE DELIVERY SYSTEMS

What is the primary reason for a surplus of hospital beds in the United States?

Insurance companies limit the length of an individual's stay

What are the primary types of hospitals?

For-profit hospitals

Not-for-profit hospitals

Long-term psychiatric care

Municipal hospitals

Veteran's administration and military hospitals

What is the role of nursing homes?

To provide long-term care, especially for individuals 65 and older

What percentage of the elderly population uses nursing home services?

5%

What is the range of costs spent on an individual that resides in a nursing home?

$35,000 to $75,000—depending upon nursing home level of care

What is the role of a hospice?

A unique type of service provided to people with advanced illnesses and limited life expectancies (< 6 months). A hospice focuses on quality-of-life issues for the terminally ill patient.

CHAPTER 25

Medical Practice: Ethical and Legal Issues

Is a physician required to have a mental or physical impairment to commit malpractice?

No. Any physician can be sued for medical malpractice.

Is malpractice a crime?

No. Malpractice is tried in civil court and may result in payment for damages inflicted.

What four elements in a malpractice case must exist in order to find liability with the treating physician (otherwise referred to as *the 4 D's*)?

Duty: There must be an established doctor-patient relationship

Deviation or dereliction: Strayed from established standard of care

Damages: Includes physical, psychological, and social ("pain and suffering")

Direct cause: Damages above must be caused directly by negligence or dereliction

How is a deviation from standard of care decided upon?

A *jury* decides if there has been a deviation from the standard of care. The jury makes this determination based upon testimony of *one or more expert witnesses* who testify as to the standard of care as generally recognized by the medical community and how the defendant deviated from that standard of care.

What is the best way to avoid a malpractice suit?

1. Maintaining your skills as a physician
2. Keeping current with the applicable standard of care
3. Maintaining a healthy physician-patient relationship

When can a physician become impaired?

When clinical judgment is affected by the following:

1. Physical illness
2. Mental illness
3. Substance abuse

Is it acceptable to work with an impaired health-care provider?

No. It is the ethical duty of a physician to report an impaired health-care provider to the proper authorities.

How does a physician's human immunodeficiency virus (HIV) status affect his or her ability to practice medicine?

Under the American Medical Association (AMA) ethical guidelines, an HIV physician should not engage in any activity that would put a patient at risk of contracting HIV (e.g., an HIV-positive surgeon may be precluded from practicing surgery. Some states require that an HIV-positive physician disclose, as part of the informed consent process, his or her HIV status before engaging in an invasive procedure that would put the patient at risk).

Is it acceptable for a physician to establish a romantic relationship with a patient or former patient?

No. It's not acceptable under any circumstances.

What is competence?

Competence is the ability to evaluate situations and make sound judgments that are:

1. Consistent throughout time
2. Consistent with the patient's belief system (except if the belief system is delusional)

Who is considered legally competent?

All adults over the age of 18 and emancipated minors—even adults with mental illness or mental retardation—unless declared incompetent by a court of law.

What is an emancipated minor?

Someone under the age of 18 who is:
1. Financially independent of his or her parents
2. Married
3. Serves in the armed forces

Note: For an unmarried minor who is not in the armed forces, many states require that the minor gets a court order declaring the minor emancipated. The court must find that the minor is financially independent and that it is in the minor's best interest to be emancipated.

Can a person be competent in some areas and not others?

Yes. Legal competence is situation specific (e.g., competence to stand trial) and can change with time. A patient can be legally competent, but not medically competent if he or she lacks the capacity to make, understand, or communicate his or her health-care decisions.

Can a physician deem a patient incompetent?

No. Legal incompetence is determined in a court of law. Any physician (not just a psychiatrist) can determine if a patient has the capacity to make medical decisions.

If a patient is ruled incompetent, how does the patient become competent again?

The case must be brought before the judge again, and after reviewing the medical evidence, the judge determines whether the patient has regained legal competence.

Who may give informed consent for a patient?

The patient *only* unless:
1. It is a bona fide emergency, and there is no one available to give consent on the patient's behalf.
2. The patient is legally incompetent (depending upon state law, the legally appointed guardian, or the agent named in a durable power of attorney for health care gives consent).
3. The patient lacks the capacity to make, understand, or communicate his or her health-care decisions (a surrogate decision-maker gives consent as

provided by state law, usually in the following order of priority: health-care agent, spouse, an adult child, parent, an adult sibling, or a grandparent).

4. The patient is a nonemancipated minor (parent or legal guardian gives consent, and in some states, someone standing in the place of a parent may also give consent).

What happens if a patient lacks the capacity to make, understand, or communicate his or her health-care decisions and has not named a health-care agent under a durable power of attorney for health-care or been appointed a legal guardian by the court?

A surrogate decision-maker may give consent on the patient's behalf and should make a good faith effort to make decisions based upon what the patient would have chosen. State law designates a list of surrogate decision-makers, usually in the following order of priority (in the absence of a health-care agent or legal guardian): spouse, adult child, parent, adult sibling, or a grandparent. State laws may differ.

What is an advance directive?

A decision made by a patient about what type of medical care he or she wishes to receive in the case that he or she is not able to make decisions in the future.

What is a durable power of attorney for health care?

A durable power of attorney for health care (or health-care proxy) is a legal document that allows the patient to designate a health-care agent to make health-care decisions on behalf of the patient when and if the patient is unable to do so. It is an advance directive.

What is a living will?

A living will is a legal document that allows a patient to decide, in advance, whether he or she wants to be kept alive by artificial means if two doctors diagnose that the patient is (1) terminally and incurably ill, (2) in a persistent vegetative state, or (3) in an irreversible coma. State laws may differ as to conditions under which a living will may be honored.

What is a DNR (do not resusicate) order?

A DNR order is an order written by a physician, after determining whether the patient is a candidate for nonresuscitation and obtaining the appropriate consent that directs medical personnel not to resuscitate a patient in the event of cardiopulmonary arrest.

When does a judge consent for medical treatment of a minor?

When a parent or legal guardian refuses to consent to medical treatment on the minor's behalf, and the physician believes that the treatment is medically necessary and justifies court intervention. A court is more likely to intervene when the proposed treatment carries a low risk and high benefit or when the minor's life is threatened.

Does this apply to a fetus?

No. The competent pregnant mother, in most circumstances, has a right to refuse any intervention on the part of the fetus even if it compromises her own or the fetus' life. In some states, courts have intervened on behalf of a viable fetus.

Under what circumstances can a nonemancipated minor receive treatment without the consent of his or her parent or legal guardian?

Although the answer is state dependent, most states allow minors to consent for treatment involving sexually transmitted diseases (STDs), contraception and pregnancy, and alcohol or illegal substance use. Some states also allow minors to consent for an abortion. Other states allow a minor to consent to an abortion, but require parental notification or a court order waiving parental notification.

When can a patient refuse treatment even though refusal is life threatening?

Anytime, as long as they have the capacity to refuse the treatment, and the refusal is an informed refusal.

Does this include artificial life support?

Yes

Is removing artificial life support the same as physician-assisted suicide?

No. Removing artificial life support is a decision that the competent, informed patient is allowed to make. It does not accelerate the natural course of the patient's disease process. Physician-assisted suicide is illegal in most states because it purposely accelerates death.

When can a physician decide to remove life support without the consent of the patient or patient's decision-maker?

A physician may remove life support without consent if the patient is legally dead. The patient must be "brain dead" in order to be declared legally dead in the United States, which includes global dysfunction of the brain (coma) and absent brainstem reflexes.

Is palliative care of the terminal patient the same as euthanasia?

No. Palliative care is not done with the intention of accelerating death. It is done with the intention of making the patient comfortable through the natural end point of a terminal illness. However, palliative care may unintentionally accelerate death as a side effect.

What is an informed consent?

Informed consent is required if the proposed treatment or procedure involves a material risk to the patient. An informed consent includes the voluntary agreement by a patient to proceed with treatment after the physician has discussed the procedure, risks, benefits, and outcome of the procedure or treatment, alternative treatments (including no treatment), and the risk, benefits, and outcomes of those alternatives.

Does consent have to be written?

No. Basic consent (e.g., consent to touching contact during a physical exam) need not be in writing and is often implied. An informed consent should be in writing and documented in the chart.

Can a physician refuse to treat patients based on race, financial status, and presence of mental illness or HIV status?

Generally, a physician may refuse to treat a patient as long as the reasons for refusal are not illegal. Illegal reasons to refuse treatment include race, national origin, gender, religion, disability (which includes mental illness and HIV status). Except in emergency situations, a physician may refuse to treat a patient based upon inability to pay.

If a patient is homicidal, is a physician allowed to break patient confidentiality?

Yes. In almost all states, the *Tarasoff* decision applies, which requires a physician to warn the person in severe danger and notify law enforcement. In states such as Georgia, *Tarasoff* has not been adopted. Instead, the physician has a duty to prevent harm by the patient if there is a right to control. In other words, if a physician has the legal right to initiate involuntarily commitment proceedings and fails to exercise this right, the physician may be held liable for harm done by the patient to third parties if the harm was foreseeable. Georgia has not specifically recognized a duty to warn, and thus, a physician may be breaching confidentiality in warning an intended victim.

In what other circumstances is a physician required to break patient confidentiality by law?

1. A patient is considered suicidal
2. Reporting child abuse, elder abuse, or domestic violence (call Child Protective Services, Adult Protective Services, or the police)
3. Court order (except to the extent the information is privileged)
4. Patient driving without cognitive abilities to do so (some states have specific procedures and forms)
5. Reporting certain infectious diseases, including HIV/acquired immunodeficiency syndrome (AIDS)

In what other circumstances can a physician breach patient confidentiality?

If the patient signs a written authorization, the physician may disclose private health information consistent with the authorization. State law may also authorize a physician to share private health information with specified people who are at risk for contracting HIV from a patient. Disclosure of this information is controlled by state law, and physicians must proceed carefully because if state law does not authorize disclosing HIV/AIDS information, the physician may be guilty of violating Health Insurance Portability and Accountability Act of 1996 (HIPAA) which may result in fines and a prison sentence.

When can a patient be "committed" or involuntarily hospitalized?

A patient who is mentally ill, an alcoholic, or a drug abuser may be involuntarily committed if the patient presents a substantial risk of imminent harm to himself or herself, or others, or if the patient is so unable to care for his or her own physical safety as to create an imminently life-endangering crisis, and the patient needs involuntary inpatient treatment.

If a patient is involuntarily hospitalized, can a physician administer any treatment they want?

No. Even an involuntarily committed patient has the right to refuse medical treatment.

How do mentally ill patients receive treatment even if they refuse treatment?

A judge can order the administration of treatment if the patient is found incompetent to refuse treatment. Also, if the patient is violent and posing an immediate, severe danger to himself or herself, or others, this is considered a medical emergency and the physician may administer treatment without the patient's consent.

CHAPTER 26

Neurochemistry in Behavioral Sciences

NEUROANATOMY

What are the two divisions of the nervous system?	Central nervous system (CNS) Peripheral nervous system (PNS)
What are the components of the CNS?	Brain Spinal cord
Which brain structures connect the cerebral hemispheres?	Corpus callosum Commissures—anterior, posterior, hippocampal, and habenular
Which hemisphere is usually the dominant hemisphere?	Left hemisphere
What is the primary role of the left hemisphere?	It governs our ability to express ourselves in language.
Which hemisphere is usually the nondominant hemisphere?	Right hemisphere
What is the primary role of the right hemisphere?	It governs perceptual functions and the analysis of space, geometrical shapes, and forms.
What are the components of the peripheral nervous system?	Nerve fibers outside the CNS including cranial nerves, spinal nerves, and peripheral ganglia
How many cranial nerves are there?	12 cranial nerves
How many spinal nerves are there?	31 pairs of spinal nerves: 8 cervical, 12 thoracic, 5 lumbar, 5 sacral, and 1 coccygeal

In which direction does the PNS carry motor and sensory information to the CNS?

Motor information—*away* from the CNS

Sensory information—*to* the CNS

What are the components of the autonomic nervous system?

Sensory neurons and motor neurons that run between the CNS (especially the *hypothalamus* and *medulla oblongata*) and various internal organs.

BRAIN LESIONS

What will be the neuropsychiatric consequences of a frontal lobe lesion?

Deficits in concentration, judgment, motivation, and orientation

Emotional changes

Personality changes

What will be the neuropsychiatric consequences of a parietal lobe lesion?

Right parietal lobe → (contralateral neglect) result in neglecting part of the body or space

Left parietal lobe → verbal deficits

What will be the neuropsychiatric consequences of a temporal lobe lesion?

Hallucinations

Memory deficits

Personality changes

What will be the neuropsychiatric consequences of a hippocampus lesion?

Bilateral damage to hippocampus leads to massive *anterograde* and some *retrograde amnesia.*

Unilateral damage of hippocampus leads to memory storage and retrieval problems.

What will be the neuropsychiatric consequences of an amygdala lesion?

Kluver-Bucy syndrome → uninhibited behavior, hyperorality, hypersexuality

What will be the neuropsychiatric consequences of a reticular system lesion?

Sleep-wake cycle changes

What will be the neuropsychiatric consequences of a basal ganglia lesion?

Tremor or other involuntary movements as seen in Parkinson's or Huntington's diseases.

What will be the neuropsychiatric consequences of a hypothalamus lesion of the ventromedial nucleus?

Decreased satiety → leads to obesity

What will be the neuropsychiatric consequences of a hypothalamus lesion of the lateral nucleus?

Decreased hunger → leads to weight loss

What will be the neuropsychiatric consequences of a hypothalamus lesion of the anterior hypothalamus?

Disturbances of parasympathetic activity

Disturbances of body cooling

What will be the neuropsychiatric consequences of a hypothalamus lesion of the posterior hypothalamus?

Disturbances of heat conservation

What will be the neuropsychiatric consequences of a hypothalamus lesion of the septate nucleus?

Change in sexual urges and emotions

What will be the neuropsychiatric consequences of a hypothalamus lesion of the suprachiasmatic lesion?

Disturbances of circadian rhythm

NEUROTRANSMITTERS

What are the four main steps involved in neurotransmitter release?

1. Presynaptic neuron stimulation
2. Neurotransmitter release
3. Neurotransmitter moves across synaptic cleft
4. Neurotransmitter acts on postsynaptic neuron receptors

What are the two different types of neurotransmitters?

Excitatory—increase neuron firing

Inhibitory—decrease neuron firing

Pre and postsynaptic receptors are made of which substance?

Protein

Which factors contribute to the magnitude of reaction neurotransmitters have on neurons?

1. Affinity of receptors
2. Number of receptors

Where are the second messengers located and what is their role in neurotransmission?

They are low-weight, *diffusible molecules* used in *signal transduction* to relay a signal within a *cell.*

What are the three major types of second-message molecules?

Hydrophobic molecules (e.g., diacylglycerol)

Hydrophilic molecules (e.g., cyclic adenosine monophosphate [cAMP])

Gases (e.g., nitric oxide [NO])

What are the three major classes of neurotransmitters?

Amino acids
Biogenic amines
Peptides

How are neurotransmitters removed from the synaptic cleft?

Reuptake by the presynaptic neuron
Degradation by enzymes (e.g., monoamine oxidase)

Table 26.1 Neurotransmitter Alterations in Psychiatric Conditions

	Alzheimer's Disease	Anxiety	Depression	Mania	Schizophrenia
Acetylcholine	↓				
Dopamine			↓	↑	↑
GABA		↓			
Norepinephrine		↑	↓		
Serotonin		↓	↓		↑

AMINES

Which amines are included in the biogenic amines, which are also called the monoamines?

Catecholamines
Ethylamines
Indolamines
Quaternary amines

What is the monoamine theory of depression?

It proposes that there is an underlying neuroanatomical basis for depression due to deficiencies of central noradrenergic and/or serotonergic systems.

Why are metabolites of monoamines measured in psychiatric studies?

They may be present in higher levels than the primary monoamines.

What type of biogenic amine is dopamine?

Catecholamine

In which psychiatric condition(s) is an altered level of dopamine evident?

Mood disorders
Parkinson's disease
Schizophrenia

How is dopamine synthesized?

By the conversion of tyrosine to dopamine by tyrosine hydroxylase

$$\text{tyrosine} \xrightarrow{\text{tyrosine hydroxylase}} \text{dopamine}$$

What is the metabolite of dopamine?

Homovanillic acid (HVA)

In which psychiatric condition(s) can there be an increased concentration of HVA?

Psychotic disorders

Schizophrenia

In which psychiatric condition(s) can there be a decreased concentration of HVA?

Alcoholism

Depression

Parkinson's disease

What type of biogenic amine is norepinephrine?

Catecholamine

What behavioral factors does norepinephrine alter?

Anxiety

Arousal

Learning

Memory

Mood

How is norepinephrine synthesized?

Dopamine is converted to norepinephrine by β-hydroxylase

$$\text{dopamine} \xrightarrow{\beta\text{-hydroxylase}} \text{norepinephrine}$$

Where are most noradrenergic neurons located in the brain?

Locus ceruleus

What are the metabolites of norepinephrine?

3-Methoxy-4-hydroxyphenylglycol (MHPG)

Vanillylmandelic acid (VMA)

In which psychiatric condition(s) can there be a decreased concentration of MHPG?

Severe depression

In which brain condition is there an increased concentration of VMA?

Pheochromocytoma → a tumor of the adrenal medulla

What type of biogenic amine is serotonin?

Indolamine

Note: Another name for serotonin is 5-hydroxytryptamine (5-HT)

What behavioral factors does serotonin alter?

Impulse control

Mood

Sleep

Sexuality

If serotonin levels are increased, which behavioral factors will be improved?	Mood Sleep
If serotonin levels are increased, which behavioral factors will be impaired?	Sexual functioning
If serotonin levels are decreased, which behavioral factors will be impaired?	Impulse control Sleep **Note:** Patient is likely to experience depression.
How is serotonin synthesized?	Tryptophan is converted to serotonin by tryptophan hydroxylase and an amino acid decarboxylase
Where are most serotoninergic cell bodies located in the brain?	Dorsal raphe nucleus
Which pharmacologic agents are used to alter the level of serotonin in the brain?	Antidepressants—e.g., selective serotonin reuptake inhibitors (SSRIs)
What is the primary metabolite of serotonin?	5-Hydroxyindoleacetic acid (5-HIAA)
In which psychiatric condition(s) is there a decreased concentration of 5-HIAA?	Alcoholism Bulimia Impulsive behavior Pyromania—uncontrollable desire to set things on fire Severe depression Tourette's syndrome Violent behavior
What type of biogenic amine is histamine?	Ethylamine **Note:** Psychoactive agents have an affect on histamine
Which pharmacologic agents block the histamine receptor?	Antipsychotic drugs Tricyclic antidepressants (TCAs)
What are side effects of the histamine receptor blockade?	Increased appetite → contributing to weight gain and obesity Sedation
What type of biogenic amine is acetylcholine (ACh)?	Quaternary amine
Where is acetylcholine normally found in the body?	Neuromuscular junctions
Which psychiatric conditions are associated with a decrease in cholinergic neurons?	Alzheimer's disease Down syndrome Movement disorders

How is acetylcholine synthesized?
Acetyl coenzyme A (CoA) and choline are converted to acetylcholine by choline acetyltransferase in cholinergic neurons

How is acetylcholine degraded?
Acetylcholine esterase (AChE) degrades acetylcholine into acetate and choline.

Which pharmacologic agents have been shown to reduce the degradation of acetylcholine?
Donepezil

Tacrine

Note: These agents can slow the progression of diseases such as Alzheimer's disease.

What are the three primary amino acid neurotransmitters?
GABA—γ-aminobutyric acid

Glutamate

Glycine

Which amino acid neurotransmitter(s) are excitatory?
Glutamate

Which amino acid neurotransmitters(s) are inhibitory?
GABA—primary inhibitory neurotransmitter

Glycine

Which pharmacologic agents alter duration and frequency of GABA?
Barbituatuates—alter *duration* of GABA

Benzodiazepines—alter *frequency* of GABA

Which neurotransmitter regulates glutamate activity?
Glycine

Which pathologic conditions may glutamate play a role in?
Cell death mechanisms

Epilepsy

Neurodegenerative diseases

Psychotic disorders (e.g., schizophrenia)

NEUROPEPTIDES

What are the two endogenous opioids?
Endorphins

Enkephalins

What behavioral factors do endogenous opioids alter?
Anxiety

Mood

Pain

Seizure activity

Temperature regulation

Which factor does endogenous opioids alter in research studies?	Placebo effects → endogenous opioids are thought to play a major role in the placebo effects seen in research studies.
Which neuropeptide(s) has been implicated in aggression and pain?	Substance P
Which neuropeptide(s) has been implicated in Alzheimer's disease?	Somatostatin Vasoactive intestinal peptide (VIP)
Which neuropeptide(s) has been implicated in mood disorders?	Oxytocin Somatostatin Substance P Vasopressin VIP
Which neuropeptide(s) has been implicated in schizophrenia?	Cholecystokinin (CCK) Neurotensin

CHAPTER 27

Epidemiology

OVERVIEW

What is the definition of epidemiology?

The study of factors that determine the frequency and distribution of disease and measure risks in human populations.

What is prevalence?

The total number of individuals who have an illness or disease in a population at a specific point in time or during a specific time frame divided by the total number of people in a population (e.g., the total number of people with breast cancer in 2006 divided by the total number of people in the population).

What is incidence?

The total number of individuals who are newly diagnosed with an illness or disease divided by the total number of individuals who are at risk of developing the disease or illness (e.g., the total number of people who are newly diagnosed with acquired immunodeficiency syndrome [AIDS] divided by the total number of people who are human immunodeficiency virus [HIV] positive).

What equation represents the relationship between prevalence and incidence?

Prevalence = incidence × disease duration → ($P = I \times DD$)
Note: This equation holds true if prevalence and incidence are stable.

What is the relationship between prevalence and incidence in chronic diseases?

Prevalence > incidence for chronic diseases (e.g., cardiovascular disease)

What is the relationship between prevalence and incidence in acute diseases?

Prevalence = incidence in acute diseases (e.g., severe acute respiratory distress syndrome [SARS])

RESEARCH STUDY DESIGNS

What are the three different types of research study designs?

Case-control

Cohort

Cross-sectional

What is a case-control study?

An observational study that compares subjects who have an illness (cases) with subjects who do not have an illness (controls).
Note: This study is often retrospective.

What is a cohort study?

An observational study that compares subjects based on the presence or absence of risk factors. This study follows subjects who are free of illness at the initiation of the study, over a period of time, for the development of disease.

What are the two types of cohort studies?

Historical

Prospective

What is a historical cohort study?

A historical cohort study is a nonconcurrent study that evaluates a cohort of individuals at different times who are not experiencing the risk factor or the treatment at the same time. (e.g., A study is constructed to evaluate whether lead exposure 5 years ago is linked to increased incidence of mental illness in 1000 men and women who went to an elementary school with toxic lead levels.)

What is a prospective cohort study?

A prospective cohort study is a concurrent study that evaluates a cohort of individuals experiencing the risk factor or the treatment at the same time. (e.g., A study is constructed to evaluate whether children exposed to secondhand smoke starting at birth will be more susceptible to lung cancer than those children not exposed to secondhand smoke starting at birth.)

What is a cross-sectional study?

An observational study that compares subjects at a specific point in time. **Note:** The subjects may or may not have an illness or disease at the time of the study.

What is a clinical trial?

An experimental cohort study in which subjects with a specific illness are given different treatments to determine their therapeutic benefit. **Note:** Some subjects in this study may be given a placebo.

What are two primary characteristics of high-quality clinical trials?

They are both randomized and double-blind.

TESTING

What are the attributes of useful testing instruments?

Lacks bias

Reliable Valid

Name the types of bias that may be prevalent in a research study.

Admission rate bias

Lead time bias

Nonresponse bias

Sampling bias

Selection bias

Which bias can occur when hospital A admits sicker patients than hospital B?

Admission rate bias

Which bias can occur when a disease or illness is detected earlier leading to increased survival time?

Lead time bias

Which bias can occur when people fail to return surveys or respond to a phone or email survey?

Nonresponse bias

Which bias can occur when a study favors selecting subjects that have a particular characteristic or set of characteristics?

Sampling bias

Which bias can occur if the subjects studied are not representative of the target population about which conclusions are drawn?

Selection bias

What percentage of patients generally respond to placebos?
Usually at least 33% of patients

What happens to the response rate to placebos in psychiatric conditions?
It increases in psychiatric illnesses.

What is the definition of a double-blind study?
A study in which neither the research scientist nor the subject knows which intervention the subject is receiving.

If initially group A receives a treatment and group B receives a placebo, and later if group A receives the placebo and group B receives a treatment, what type of research study is being utilized?
Crossover studies

What is reliability?
It is the reproducibility of a given test.

What type of reliability is demonstrated when different examiners are able to achieve test results that are similar?
Interrater reliability

What type of reliability is demonstrated when subsequent tests yield similar results to initial tests?
Test-retest reliability

What is the definition of validity?
It determines whether a test measures what it is supposed to measure.

What is the definition of precision?
It is the consistency and reproducibility of a test.
Note: There should not be any random variation.

What is the definition of accuracy?
It determines how true test measurements are.

		Disease +	Disease −
Exposure	+	a	b
	−	c	d

What is the sensitivity of a test?
It is the ability to detect a disease or illness.

How is sensitivity calculated?
True positives divided by all of the individuals with a disease or illness

Sensitivity = $a/(a + c)$

What is the specificity of a test?

It is the ability to detect health in an individual.

How is specificity calculated?

True negatives divided by all of the people without a disease or illness

Specificity = $d/(b + d)$

What is positive predictive value (PPV)?

If there is a positive test, it is the likelihood of disease or illness.

How is positive predictive value calculated?

True positives divided by all people with a positive test

PPV = $a/(a + b)$

What is negative predictive value (NPV)?

If there is a negative test, it is the likelihood of health.

How is negative predictive value calculated?

True negatives divided by all people with a negative test

NPV = $d/(c + d)$

If the prevalence of a disease or illness in a population is low, what happens to the positive predictive value?

There is a low positive predictive value.

If the prevalence of a disease is high, what happens to the positive predictive value and negative predictive value?

↑ positive predictive value

↓ negative predictive value

What is the definition of clinical probability?

It is the likelihood that an event will occur.

What is the definition of attack rate?

It is the type of incidence rate which is utilized to describe disease outbreaks.

How is the attack rate calculated?

Number of individuals with a disease or illness during the study period divided by the number of individuals at risk of developing the disease or illness.

If 2 out of 100 people who are exposed to anthrax spores develop malignant pustules, what is the attack rate of anthrax?

2%

MEASURES OF ASSOCIATION

Which measures are used to quantify risks in population studies?

Attributable risk

Odds ratio

Relative risk

Which measure(s) of association is used to evaluate cohort studies?

Attributable risk

Relative risk

Note: These risks are evaluated in prospective data.

Which measure(s) of association is used to evaluate case-control studies?

Odds ratio

Note: The odds ratio is evaluated in retrospective data.

What is the definition of attributable risk (AR)?

AR is used to determine how much credit a risk factor should be given for causing a disease or illness (e.g., how likely is a high cholesterol diet to lead to atherosclerosis?).

How is AR calculated?

AR determines the disease rate in exposed subjects minus that in unexposed subjects.

$([a/(a + b)] - [c/(c + d)])$

If the incidence rate of atherosclerosis in the general population in Atlanta, GA is 10/100 and in individuals with a high cholesterol diet is 50/100, what is the attributable risk?

40/100 → This answer assumes that there is a properly matched control.

What is relative risk (RR)?

RR determines the ratio of disease rate in exposed subjects to that in subjects who are unexposed.

$([a/(a + b)] \ / \ [c/(c + d)])$

When is RR clinically significant?

If RR is not equal to 1, it is not clinically significant.

If the RR is greater than 1, what can be said about the risk?

There is an increased risk of the disease or illness.
Note: If the RR < 1, there is a decreased risk of illness or disease.

What is an odds ratio (OR)?

This determines the relative risk if the prevalence of disease is low.

$OR = ad/bc$

What would be concluded about a study if the 95% confidence interval for RR or OR includes 1?

The study would be inconclusive.

CHAPTER 28

Biostatistics

STATISTICAL DISTRIBUTION

What are the three measures of central tendency?

Mean

Median

Mode

What is the definition of mean?

It is the average of a set of numbers.

What is the definition of median?

It is the middle number in a set of numbers when they are put in sequential order.
Note: If there is an even data set, the median is the average of the two middle values in the data set.

What is the definition of mode?

It is the number that appears most frequently in a set of numbers.

Using the following set of numbers, what are the mean, median, and mode? 1, 2, 3, 4, 5, 6, 7, 8, 9, 10, 11, 12, 12

Mean = [(1 + 2 + 3 + 4 + 5 + 6 + 7 + 8 + 9 + 10 + 11 + 12 + 12)/13] = 90/13 = 6.923
Median = 7
Mode = 12

What is the range of a data set?

The difference between the highest and lowest values in a data set.
Note: The range in the data set above is 12 − 1 = 11.

Define normal distribution.

A set of numbers in which the mean, median, and mode are equal.
Mean = median = mode

What type of curve demonstrates a normal distribution?

Gaussian or bell-shaped curve

When a data set shows a large number of high values and a small number of low values, what is the distribution of the data set?

Negatively skewed
Mean < median < mode
Note: The tail of the curve is on the left or on the negative end of the number line.

When a data set shows a large number of low values and a small number of high values, what is the distribution of the data set?

Positively skewed
Mean > median > mode
Note: The tail of the curve is on the right or on the positive end of the number line.

When a data set shows two humps, what is the distribution of the data set?

Bimodal

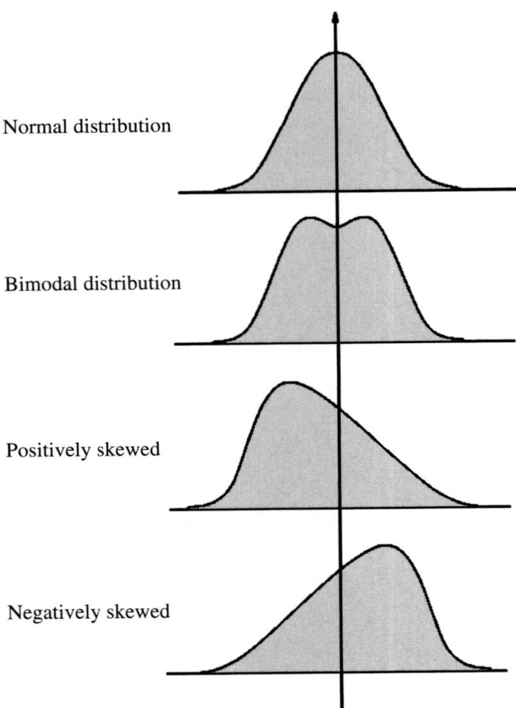

Fig. 28.1 Statistical Frequency Distributions.

What is a variable?

It is a quantity that changes throughout time.

What is an independent variable?

It is an attribute that the research scientist may adjust in an experiment.

What is a dependent variable?

It is the outcome associated with an experimental adjustment.

What is the correlation coefficient (r)?

It expresses the strength of a relationship between two variables. Its value must be between the values of −1.0 and +1.0.
Note: The (−) sign implies a negative correlation and the (+) sign implies a positive correlation.

Why is it important to take the absolute value of the r?

The absolute value of r will determine the strength of the correlation.

What is the definition of standard deviation (σ)?

It is the *root mean square* deviation from the average. The standard deviation is defined as the *square root* of the *variance*. It is the most frequently used measure to determine statistical dispersion.

How is σ calculated?

1. Square each deviation from the mean in a data set
2. Add the squared deviations
3. Divide by the number of values in the data set minus 1
4. Calculate the square root of result

What percentage of the population falls in 1 standard deviation from the mean?

68%

What percentage of the population falls in 2 standard deviations from the mean?

95%

What percentage of the population falls in 3 standard deviations from the mean?

99.7%

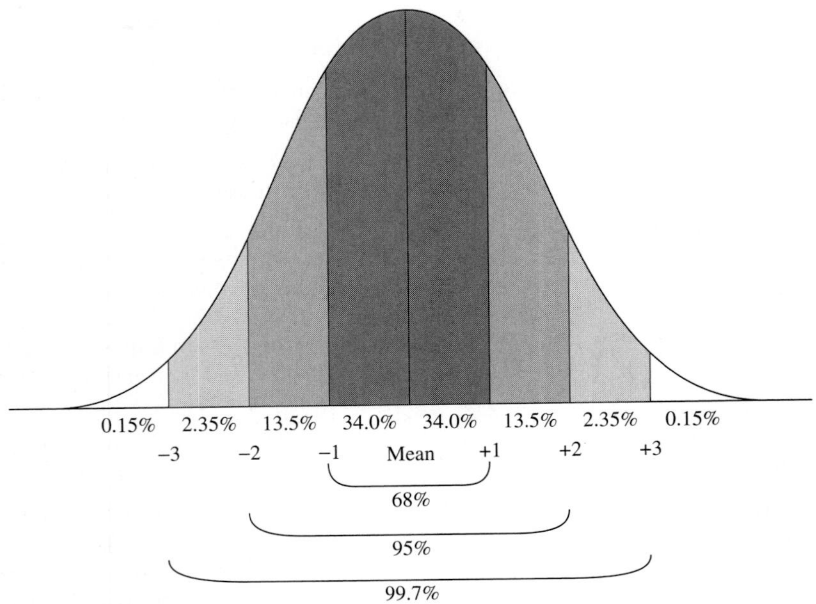

Fig. 28.2 Normal (Gaussian) Distribution Represented by a Bell-Shaped Curve. The (+) and (–) numbers under the curve correspond to the standard deviations from the mean.

What is the standard error of the mean (SEM)?

SEM = standard deviation (σ)/ √sample size (n) SEM = $\sigma/\sqrt{n}$

Given the following data set (4, 5, 7, 8), what is the mean, σ, and SEM?

$$4 + 5 + 7 + 8 = 24$$

$$24/4 = 6 \rightarrow \text{mean}$$

$$(4-6)^2 + (5-6)^2 + (7-6)^2 + (8-6)^2 = \sqrt{10}/(4-1) = \sqrt{10}/3 \rightarrow \sigma$$

$$(\sqrt{10}/3)/(\sqrt{4}) \rightarrow \text{SEM}$$

What is the standard normal variable?

It is the difference between an individual variable and the population mean.

How is the standard normal variable computed?

It is the z score which is computed as follows:

$$z = \frac{\text{(score in a data set)} - \text{(the mean score in a data set)}}{\text{(the standard deviation of the distribution)}}$$

What is the confidence interval (CI)?

It is an estimated range of values which is likely to include an unknown population parameter, the estimated range being calculated from a given set of sample data.
Note: The 95% CI is most frequently used → the associated z score is $z = 1.96$

How is the CI calculated?

$CI = \text{mean} \pm z\ (\sigma/\sqrt{n})$

STATISTICAL HYPOTHESIS AND ERROR TYPES

What is the null hypothesis (H_0)?

It is the hypothesis that indicates that there is no difference between two groups or that the experimental intervention does not have an effect on the treatment group.
Note: At the beginning of an experimental study, the researcher decides whether or not to accept or reject the null hypothesis.

What is the alternative hypothesis (H_1)?

It is the hypothesis that indicates that there is a difference between two groups or that the experimental intervention does have an effect on the treatment group.

What is a type I (α) error?

A type I error occurs when the null hypothesis is rejected and it is indeed correct. This occurs when a research scientist states that the experimental intervention had an effect when it really did not.

What is a type II (β) error?

A type II error occurs when the null hypothesis is not rejected and it is indeed incorrect. This occurs when a research scientist states that the experimental intervention did not have an effect when it really did.

What is power?

It is the probability of rejecting the null hypothesis when it is indeed incorrect.

Which equation is used to determine power?

Power = $1-\beta$.

If the sample size increases, what happens to power? It increases

What value of power is considered acceptable in research? Power > 0.8

What is the probability (*p*) value? It determines the random error of an experiment or the percent chance that an experiment conclusion was derived from chance alone. It determines the chance of a type I error occurring.

What *p* value is most commonly considered a cutoff to determine statistical significance? $p < 0.05$.
If $p < 0.05$, the research scientist can reject the null hypothesis.

STATISTICAL TESTS

What type of statistical tests is used to evaluate statistical significance between groups when there is a normal distribution of values? Parametric statistical tests

What are the examples of parametric statistical tests?
t-test
Analysis of variance (ANOVA)
Linear correlation

What type of statistical tests is used to evaluate statistical significance between groups when there is not a normal distribution of values? Nonparametric statistical tests

What are the examples of nonparametric statistical tests?
Kruskal-Wallis
Mann-Whitney
Wilcoxon's

What type of statistical tests is used to compare proportions or analyze categorical data? Categorical tests

What is an example of a categorical test? Chi-square also called Fisher exact test

What type of parametric statistical test determines the difference between the means of two groups? *t*-test

Which type of *t*-test evaluates the means of two groups at one period of time? Independent (nonpaired) *t*-test (e.g., comparing the mean income of one set of orthopaedic surgeons,

Group Bone, to the mean income of another set of orthopaedic surgeons, Group Tendon, at the beginning of the calendar year).

Which type of *t*-test evaluates the means of two groups at two different time periods?

Dependent (paired) *t*-test (e.g., comparing the mean income of one set of orthopaedic surgeons, Group Bone, to the mean income of another set of orthopaedic surgeons, Group Tendon, at the beginning and in the middle of the calendar year).

Which type of parametric statistical test determines the difference of means of more than two groups?

ANOVA

Which type of ANOVA test determines the difference of means of more than two groups using only one variable?

One-way ANOVA (e.g., comparing the mean income of orthopaedic surgeons in Group Bone, Group Tendon, and Group Ligament at the beginning of the calendar year).

Which type of ANOVA test determines the difference of means of more than two groups using two variables?

Two-way ANOVA (e.g., comparing the mean income and malpractice insurance rate of orthopaedic surgeons in Group Bone, Group Tendon, and Group Ligament at the beginning of the calendar year).

Which type of parametric statistical test determines the relation between two continuous variables?

Linear correlation

What types of data are evaluated in statistical tests?

Nominal

Ordinal

Interval

Ratio

What is nominal data?

It is categorical data where the order of the categories is arbitrary (e.g., gender, religious beliefs).

What is ordinal data?

It is categorical data where there is a logical ordering to the categories (e.g., first place winner, second place winner, third place winner, and so forth).

What is interval data?

It is continuous data where differences are interpretable, but where there is no "natural" zero (e.g., Celsius, Fahrenheit).

What is ratio data?	It is continuous data where both differences and ratios are interpretable. Ratio data has a natural zero (e.g., weight, height, blood pressure).
What type(s) of statistical tests would be used to evaluate nominal data?	Chi-square test
What type(s) of statistical test would be used to evaluate ordinal data?	Chi-square test
What type(s) of statistical test would be used to evaluate interval data?	*t*-tests ANOVA Linear correlation
What type(s) of statistical test would be used to evaluate ratio data?	*t*-tests ANOVA Linear correlation

CHAPTER 29

Clinical Vignettes—USMLE Style Questions

QUESTIONS AND ANSWERS

1. **A distressed mother comes to you with her 6-month-old boy, for his checkup. The child appears well-nourished and healthy. While taking the history, the mother tells you that he was born at 30 weeks, when she was 15 years old. He used to eat well, gain weight, coo, and reach for objects. However, she is worried that he is now unresponsive and silent. She has not spent any time with him since she has been devoting most of her time to her friends at school. On most occasions, she leaves him at home without anyone to care for him. On physical examination and record reviews, the child was in the 55th percentile on the growth charts at 4 months but is currently in the 15th percentile. At 4 months of age, the Moro, palmar, and stepping reflexes were present but no rooting reflex. Now at 6 months, the Moro, palmar, stepping, and rooting reflexes are all present. What do you suspect of this child?**

   The child is suffering from anaclitic depression and is showing failure to thrive.

2. **Tom and Tammy have a 4-year-old girl, Taylor, and a boy, Travis, who just turned 2. When Taylor was 2, she could walk upstairs, throw balls, ride a tricycle, follow commands, speak understandably, and went to playgroup where she played with other kids. Tom and Tammy are**

   Tammy developed within the normal time frame for a 2-year-old and Travis is also developing in a normal time frame.

concerned because all Travis does at play group is play next to the other kids. Travis runs but doesn't climb the stairs like Taylor did, he can build towers but not like Taylor did, and the parents can understand him when he speaks but their friends have a hard time. They are concerned about Travis' development since he is not as fast a learner like Taylor was. What do you tell them?	
3. A 32-year-old married woman develops hallucination and delusions 2 weeks after the delivery of a healthy baby boy. She informs the physician that she has had thoughts about harming the infant. The physician decides to hospitalize the mother immediately and place her on antipsychotic medication. What postpartum reaction has the woman experienced?	Postpartum psychosis
4. A 49-year-old male lawyer decides that he is ready for a career change. He needs a new challenge in his life to reclaim his youthfulness. He decides to open a motorcycle shop since he has always loved racing his Harley-Davidson. What emotional response is this man exhibiting at this stage of his life?	Midlife crisis
5. An 86-year-old man lost his spouse 6 months ago and recently has experienced difficulty with bookkeeping and preparing his meals. His daughter has mentioned inviting him to come and live with her. Based on common psychiatric problems that elderly face, what is this patient most likely going through?	Bereavement
6. A 66-year-old man was recently forced to resume his position as a cashier, after retiring 2 years ago, due to difficulty in paying his bills that his social security did not accommodate for. He has no children and has never been married. Which Erickson's stage of life is this man most likely experiencing?	Ego integrity vs. despair

Questions 7 to 10 correspond to the following vignette.

Bob is a medical student with obsessive-compulsive personality disorder. Which defense mechanism is he using in the scenarios below?

7. Bob was pimped excessively by Professor *Hee-Haytes*. Bob later tells his fellow medical students that Professor *Hee-Haytes* is "great!"	Reaction formation
8. Bob keeps a straight face as he discusses a tragic event he witnessed in the ER.	Isolation of affect
9. Bob's dog dies. When he is consoled by fellow students, he states "He was really old and I was expecting him to go soon anyway. Most large dogs only live until they are 10."	Intellectualization
10. Bob fails the last anatomy exam after he studied 12 hours per day in the corner of the library for 1 month. He tells his friend, "I think I failed because I didn't study enough. Besides, I am not really going to use anatomy later on."	Rationalization
11. A 41-year-old Black male is admitted to the neurology unit after a large cerebrovascular accident (CVA) in his frontal lobe. The patient is rude and constantly berates the neurology staff, including the treating team. The team decides to discharge him without proper placement in a facility that can cater to the patient's needs, justifying these actions because the patient "is a jerk." What is this scenario an example of?	Countertransference
12. Psychiatry is consulted on a 39-year-old White female because the staff cannot agree on a correct treatment plan and is constantly fighting with each other. Some of the staff members believe this patient is "a nightmare" while the others describe her as "an angel." The psychiatry resident reviews the records to find that this patient has a	Splitting

long history of borderline personality disorder. What defense mechanism utilized unconsciously by this patient resulted in this confusing scenario?	
13. A 2-year-old has come to visit you for his well-child check. As you are talking to his mom, he starts to hit, scream, and cry when not allowed to climb on furniture. The mother asks you for behavioral assistance. What is your best response?	Ignore the tantrum
14. A 15-year-old is undergoing chemotherapy for Ewing's sarcoma. He has received four sessions of chemotherapy at the children's hospital which is decorated with sports murals. One day while shopping with his mother, he sees a large sports drawing and suddenly experiences severe nausea and vomiting. What best describes this reaction?	Classical conditioning

The next two questions (items 15 and 16) correspond to the following vignette.

A 19-year-old college student is brought to the ER by his fraternity brothers at 3 A.M. after a Friday night party. The young man is arousable to painful stimuli only, his vitals signs are temperature 100.4°F, heart rate (HR) 115, blood pressure (BP) 135/70, respiratory rate (RR) 9. His pupils are 1 mm and reactive. His friends have no idea what he has taken, but they admit that alcohol and other drugs were available at the party.

15. What drug has the patient most likely ingested?	Alcohol
16. What drug should be administered immediately after this patient arrives in the ER?	Naloxone
17. A 24-year-old female at 21 weeks gestation comes to the ER requesting treatment for her addiction to oxyContin (oxycodone). You are sent to the ER to evaluate the patient and determine what course of treatment should be pursued. What are the treatment options for this patient?	Detoxification and rehabilitation

18. A young woman presents to your office and says she thinks she is having psychiatric problems. She reluctantly reports that she has had a number of disturbingly vivid hallucinations, usually right before she falls asleep and has even had the frightening experience of waking up seemingly paralyzed. On further questioning, she notes that she frequently falls asleep suddenly during the day, and fell to the floor when her friends shouted "surprise" at her last birthday party. What is the best treatment?	Start a stimulant
19. An 83-year-old woman presents to your office because she feels as though she is spending less time getting a restful sleep at night. She has heard from her friends that there are changes in sleep that occur with aging. What stage of sleep is associated with an increase in blood pressure and pulse and tends to decrease with age?	Rapid eye movement (REM) sleep
20. A 19-year-old male is brought to the emergency room by his college roommate for delusions, hallucinations, and disorganized speech that has occurred for the last 7 months. He is concerned about his roommate because he does not seem like his normal self. The roommate is concerned that the patient may have schizophrenia. The patient's father was diagnosed with schizophrenia at age 22. What is the likelihood of a first-degree relative of a proband (affected individual) developing schizophrenia?	10%
21. A 41-year-old Down syndrome patient has had a gradual deterioration in cognitive functioning. Lately, she has been unable to remember her home address, and her daughter has noticed that she has difficulty remembering names of people she has known throughout the duration of her life. Her primary care	Chromosome 21

physician diagnoses her with Alzheimer's disease. Which chromosome has been found to be defective in these patients?

22. **You are the third year medical student on the psychiatry consult service. You and your resident are called to the ER for a patient who was recently admitted to the inpatient psychiatry service for depression and suicidal ideation. While in the hospital, he complained of having trouble sleeping and was given something to help both his depression and sleep problems. The patient received a prescription for this medication when he was discharged from the service 2 days ago. He now presents to the ER with a 3-hour history of a painful erection. What drug was the patient given?** Trazodone

Questions 23 to 25 correspond to the following vignette.

A 26-year-old female presents to your clinic with complaints of episodes of shortness of breath, palpitations, tingling around her mouth, and blurry vision. She has only experienced two of these episodes, but she fears that she may have more. She asks you to start her on some medication to help with these fears and the episodes themselves. Her last menstrual period was 7 weeks ago, and she has a history of cocaine abuse when she was a teenager.

23. **What class of medication would be most useful in providing immediate relief of symptoms for this patient?** Benzodiazepine

24. **Why might this class of medications be contraindicated in this patient?** She may be pregnant

25. **What is a possible alternative?** Buspirone

26. **A 21-year-old White male is referred to you after he was released from a local psychiatric hospital, where he was diagnosed with schizophrenia. Apparently, he was a college student, but 3 years ago he began to withdraw socially and lost motivation. More recently he became increasingly disorganized and bizarre. During the last 3 years he has also had several bouts of major depression. What is a positive feature of his presentation?** Significant depressive episodes

27. **Being a top-notch medical student, a friend asks your opinion about his grandmother. She is in her mid-seventies and has started to develop some paranoid behaviors over the last 2 years. Your friend reports that she has never had anything like this before, but has been more forgetful lately. The family is very afraid that she has schizophrenia. What would the best response be?**	This is unlikely to be schizophrenia due to her age and lack of prior psychiatric symptoms.
28. **A 27-year-old African American man is brought to the ER by police because he was running naked around his neighborhood. During your interview the patient keeps talking continuously, is mostly cursing you and the police, cannot focus on the interview, is loud and difficult to redirect. Patient is pacing up and down in the interview room. What is the substance that you expect to find in his urine toxicology screen?**	Cocaine
29. **A 47-year-old-White woman presents to your office with a long history of major depressive disorder complaining of blurred vision and episodes of dizziness. What is the antidepressant that this patient is most likely taking?**	Amitriptyline
30. **An 85-year-old woman with a history of Alzheimer's disease is brought to the ER by her family for new onset hallucinations. She is initially cooperative with the interview, but easily distracted, and eventually dozes off. The family tells you that she started acting confused, and easily agitated last night. This morning she initially seemed fine, but later began seeing people who weren't there. What is the most likely diagnosis?**	Delirium
31. **A 57-year-old man with a history of hepatitis C, end-stage liver disease, and peptic ulcers underwent surgery to repair a perforated ulcer 2 days ago. He is agitated, confused, and he believes bugs are crawling on him. He appears floridly**	Alcohol withdrawal

delirious and you begin his workup. His blood work reveals no evidence of infection, his blood pressure is becoming more labile, and heart rate is increasing. Your attending physician shows up and is very concerned that he may seize. What is the most likely etiology for the delirium?

32. **A 35-year-old female is rushed to the ER after sustaining minor injuries from a motor vehicle accident. During the interview, you ask her what happened. She states "I lost control of my car. I was rushing to pick my teenage daughter up from band practice and I hate to have her waiting. It's so dangerous for children out there and I'm worried some stranger may kidnap her." She then admits to speeding but says she left work late because she had to double check her secretary's work because "you can't trust everyone." Her husband arrives soon after and says "Doc, could you give my wife something for her nerves? She's always so high strung and worrying about everything. I can't even buy a pack of gum without her thinking we won't have enough money to pay the bills." What is this patient's most likely diagnosis?**

Generalized anxiety disorder (GAD)

33. **An 18-year-old male comes to the clinic for an acute visit. He recently enlisted in the military and has since noted increased urgency and frequency of urination. This is the second time in 3 months that you have treated him for a urinary tract infection (UTI) and you are beginning to become suspicious of a chronic condition. He denies having any history of UTIs before his enlistment and also denies any sexual activity. You then ask "How many times per day do you urinate?" He replies, "I usually go once or twice. Since I've been in basic training I'm not alone often and I'm just not**

Social phobia

comfortable with the community restroom thing." He proceeds to tell you how uncomfortable he is using the restroom while others are around. He states "I know its silly but I get all nervous and keep thinking all eyes are on me whenever other people are in the restroom. But it's ok because I normally just hold it until I'm alone." What is his most likely psychiatric diagnosis?

34. A 12-year-old girl and her parents present to your office with a chief complaint of dysphagia for 3 days. According to the girl's parents, who are very concerned and anxious, the girl choked while eating lunch 3 days ago and the Heimlich maneuver was performed to expel the food. Since then she has been unable to swallow any solids or liquids. Additionally, she is unable to swallow any of her normal oral secretions, and has been spitting constantly in a container. On exam, the girl is very quiet, calm, and somewhat unconcerned about her condition. Assuming physical exam is normal and an upper gastrointestinal (GI) series fails to reveal any pathology, what is the likely diagnosis?

Conversion disorder

35. A 25-year-old nursing student presents to your office as a patient for the first time with a chief complaint of hematuria. Physical exam is benign, and a basic lab workup is unremarkable except for the urinalysis which demonstrates a large number of red blood cells (RBCs). You admit her to the hospital service for a workup of her hematuria, and you decide to look through her medical record for any clues toward the etiology of her hematuria. You discover that she has seen multiple physicians for similar complaints, all of which were extensively evaluated, and revealed no source of pathology. You become suspicious of which psychiatric disorder?

Factitious disorder

36. A young woman is sitting alone in a bar. She does not speak to anyone else in the bar all night and just sits on the stool watching others and drinking her beer. The next day in her therapy session, she tells you about the previous night. She says there were several people she would have liked to talk to in the bar, but they just would not have been interested in her. In addition to therapy, what could be added to her treatment regimen to help with this disorder?

Assertiveness training

37. On your gynecology rotation, you and your resident are called to the ER to evaluate a woman with vaginal bleeding. When you get to the ER the resident recognizes the patient's name and dumps her off on you saying he will be back in a few minutes to check up on you. When you enter the room you notice a rather pleasant woman sitting on a stretcher. You introduce yourself, and she says "I am so happy you will be my doctor! You really know what you are doing, not like the idiots at the other hospital across town." During your exam you notice multiple scars on the woman wrists and forearms. What is this woman exhibiting characteristics of?

Splitting

38. A 21-year-old woman presents with an inability to recall any events associated with an explosion in her college dormitory in which a number of her college classmates were killed. She does not report any other memory loss other than that concerning the explosion in her dormitory. Which disorder is this patient suffering from?

Dissociative amnesia

39. A 42-year-old presents to his primary-care physician and reports that he has had multiple episodes of perceiving objects in his environment as much larger than they really are. He also states that he feels detached from his body at times. The patient states that he is aware that these are only perceptions and not reality. What is he suffering from?	Depersonalization disorder
40. A 39-year-old woman sends her 17-year-old daughter to your office because she has become more irritable over the last 4 months. You enter the room and find a young woman dressed in a large sweatshirt and baggy jeans sitting slouched in a chair. When you ask her about her mother's concerns, she smiles and says that her mother is overreacting and that she is just stressed out because she is in the middle of applying to 6 Ivy League colleges and is currently the captain of the swim team. On exam, she is 5 ft 8 in. tall and weighs 104 lb. Physical exam is completely normal. What is the best treatment of the condition this patient is exhibiting?	Hospitalization
41. A 45-year-old woman comes to your office for a regular health-maintenance visit. Near the end of the visit she looks at you and asks if you know of any good diets as she would like to drop a few pounds. She is currently 1.4 m tall and weighs 63 kg. What is her BMI?	32
42. A 14-year-old male is brought to a psychiatrist because of his disregard for rules set by authority figures at home and in school. He has set numerous fires in his neighborhood. His parents are concerned that he seems to have no regard for the feelings of others. Which disorder is this patient most likely to be diagnosed with?	Conduct disorder

43. A 3-year-old girl presents with problems forming social relationships. She engages in repetitive behavior, and she has a strong interest in learning all about the different types of bubble gum in the world. Her mother states that the girl has not had any cognitive deficits and has had no developmental language delay. Which condition is the patient most likely to be diagnosed with?	Asperger's disorder
44. Mr. A presents to your office for follow-up for asthma. He admits that he has been drinking more over the last couple of weeks. You ask about his mood and he answers "so-so" but admits to more frustration and irritability, no energy, and decreased sexual desire for his wife of thirty years. What is the next best question that you should ask Mr. A?	"Have you had any thoughts about death or hurting yourself?"
45. Ms. B is an eager ballerina who presents to the ER while you are on duty. She drove herself to the hospital and states that due to gaining weight she was not selected as prima ballerina in a new production. Upon questioning, she shows you several small lacerations on her left wrist. She also discloses that she has been feeling more depressed with poor appetite, no energy, and increasing hopelessness. She discloses that she lives alone and has never seen a psychiatrist. As part of your treatment management, what is the best next step?	Encourage hospitalization for stabilization of her crisis.
46. A 20-year-old college student goes to her university's career center to take an objective test to determine career-counseling recommendations? Which personality test did she take?	Minnesota Multiphasic Personality Inventory
47. A second grade boy is being evaluated for mental retardation based upon his teacher's recommendation. His teacher has noticed that the boy has significantly impaired intellectual abilities compared to his classmates. Which test should be given to determine if this boy has mental retardation?	Stanford-Binet scale

48. A 32-year-old male who is happily married does not become sexually aroused unless his wife wears a specific black negligee. He has always had an obsession with objects to give him sexual gratification. Which sexual paraphilia does this patient have?	Fetishism
49. A 25-year-old female experiences intense painful vaginal spasms whenever she goes to get a pelvic examination and engages in sexual intercourse. She has begun psychological counseling to treat her condition. Which type of sexual dysfunction does she suffer from?	Vaginismus
50. A 21-year-old female college student decides to go on a date with her boyfriend of 2 years. They decide to go out dancing, and she consumes a large volume of alcohol while out. When they return to her dorm room, the boyfriend decides to ask the girlfriend is she wants to have sex. Since they had had sex before, he coerces her to have sex citing their long-term relationship shows his commitment to her. She half-heartedly agrees before passing out. The boyfriend decides to have sex with her since she indicated it was alright with her. Would the incident that occurred be considered a sexual assault and why?	Yes, the female college student experienced numerous types of forces in that she was under the influence of alcohol and coercion when she consented to have sex.
51. A 32-year-old female has three children. As a single mother, she has struggled to take care of herself and her children. She frequently finds herself not having the resources to obtain basic necessities for her family including food and clothing. Her children are afraid of her because she physically abuses them on a regular basis. Which trait of child abusers is most evident in the woman in this scenario?	Low socioeconomic status

52. **You are seeing an 80-year-old patient with hyperlipidemia and hypertension for follow-up treatment. He is taking several "state-of-the-art," newly released medications. There is no overall improvement in the patient's conditions since his initial intake. Following further discussion, you find that he is only taking his medications on Monday, Wednesday, and Friday because the medications are too expensive. What do you tell this patient to increase his compliance?**

"The newer medications can sometimes be very expensive. Let's discuss which other medications you might be able to afford to take everyday."

53. **A 45-year-old male with chronic pain is requesting his practicing registered nurse (PRN) pain medications as often as he can. What is the most likely explanation?**

The patient's pain regimen is inadequate

54. **A 35-year-old high school teacher has recently begun working at a school with more health-care plan options than his prior place of employment. He is excited about the possibility of choosing a plan with low premiums. He also would like the option of having some flexibility with the type of plan he chooses. What plan is the best option for him to choose?**

Point-of-service (POS) plan

55. **A U. S. senator is considering proposing changes to current Medicare guidelines because she feels as though not all groups of people receive the same benefits due to differences in life expectancies for different segments of the population. Which group of people is least likely to receive benefits of the Medicare program?**

Black men

56. **Bob is a third year medical student. His third year medical school colleague is a substance abuser and sometimes comes to the wards stoned. Who does Bob report this to?**

Medical school dean

57. Bob is a single medical student rotating in ophthalmology. He is particularly attracted to Miss B, a patient, who expressed a similar attraction to him. Bob completes his ophthalmology rotation in 4 days. What response is the best way to handle this situation?

Since we have worked so hard to establish a physician-patient relationship that has helped you recover, establishing a romantic relationship would impede your ability to return to see me as a physician both now and in the future.

58. A 76-year-old woman presents to the ER after experiencing a cerebrovascular accident. She is still able to communicate very well with the physicians, but it is clear that she has neglected the entire left side of her body. She is well-groomed on the right side, but her face, hair, clothes, and shoes are disheveled on the left side of her body. This woman experienced a lesion to what portion of the brain?

Right parietal lobe

59. A 56-year-old man presents to his primary care physician with signs of depression. After taking a thorough history and physical exam, the physician diagnoses him with severe depression and starts him on a prescription of fluoxetine, a selective serotonin reuptake inhibitor (SSRI). Which metabolite profile is likely to be present in this patient?

3-Methoxy-4-hydroxyphenylglycol

60. A biomedical researcher conducts a retrospective study to evaluate whether or not high sun exposure is linked to skin cancer. She interviews 100 patients to determine the extent of their sun exposure over their lifetime. Fifty patients were selected because they had skin cancer. The other 50 patients were selected randomly. Here are the results:

		Skin cancer +	Skin cancer –
High sun exposure	+	45	15
	–	5	35

What is the odds ratio?

(45 × 35)/(15 × 5)

61. After a meta-analysis of studies evaluating the likelihood cigarette smokers will develop lung cancer, it is determined that 75% of all persons who smoke will develop lung cancer. If two individuals smoke, what is the likelihood that at least one individual will develop lung cancer?

93.75%

62. A medical research scientist has been working fervently to develop a pharmaceutical intervention to deal with the problem of obesity in the United States. She has developed a drug called GJCHS-1 and tested it on 200 people with a body mass index (BMI) of greater than 30. She decides to complete a double-blind randomized study in which patients are placed in either group 1 or group 2. Each group contained 100 patients. At the beginning of the study, the baseline BMI was recorded for all patients enrolled in the study. Group 1 received the placebo and group 2 received the treatment drug, GJCHS-1. If after the drug trial is completed, the medical research scientist reports a *p* value of < 0.02, what should the researcher decide about the experimental results with regards to the null hypothesis and statistical significance? Note the experimental results below.

Reject the null hypothesis and the results are statistically significant

	Group 1 (placebo)	Group 2 (GJCHS-1)
Initial BMI (average)	38	40
BMI after 21 days (average)	36	29

63. A research scientist would like to evaluate the racial profile of the residents in two orthopaedic surgery residency programs. She believes that residency program A has a significantly larger representation of underrepresented minorities than residency program B. Each resident is asked to indicate whether they are Caucasian, African American, Hispanic, Asian or Pacific Islander, or other. Which statistical test would be most useful in sorting through the data provided?	Chi-square test

Suggested Readings

Anderson N, Black D. *Introductory Textbook of Psychiatry. 3rd ed.*, Washington, DC: American Psychiatry Publishing: 2000.

Fadem B. *Behavioral Science in Medicine*. Baltimore, MD: Lippincott Williams & Wilkins, 2004.

National Institute of Neurological Disorders and Stroke, part of National Institutes of Health Web site. Available at:
http://www.ninds.nih.gov/disorders/tourette/detail_tourette. htm#56653231. Accessed 2/15/06.

Index

Page numbers followed by italic *f* or *t* refer to figures or tables, respectively.